15-Minute Daily Chair Yoga for Beginners and Seniors

Empower Your Body and Mind: Gentle Routines for Strength, Flexibility, and Inner Peace at Any Age

Tessa Linden

Table of Content

Author's Note

Dear Reader,

As I sit down to write this note, I can't help but feel a sense of gratitude and fulfillment. This book, like chair yoga itself, is a labor of love—a product of my passion for movement, wellness, and helping others discover their own strength and peace, no matter where they are in life.

I wrote this book because I believe everyone deserves to feel empowered in their body. Chair yoga has a unique ability to bridge the gap for those who feel that traditional exercise isn't accessible. It's not just about poses; it's about the possibility of rediscovering joy in movement, finding stillness in breath, and reconnecting with yourself in ways that are healing and profound.

As a lifelong advocate for mindful living, I've seen firsthand how small changes can transform lives. I've met seniors who regained independence, individuals recovering from injuries who found hope, and beginners who surprised themselves with how much they could achieve. I wanted to bring these possibilities to you, in the simplest and most supportive way possible.

This isn't just a guide to exercises; it's an invitation to a lifestyle. Whether you're seeking strength, flexibility, relaxation, or just a moment of peace in your day, this book was designed with you in mind. It's meant to inspire, motivate, and empower you, no matter your starting point.

Writing this book wasn't without its challenges. Translating physical movements into clear and accessible words required deep thought and care. I aimed to create a resource that feels like a supportive friend, guiding you step by step. However, I know no book is perfect. If you come across any errors or unclear instructions, I humbly ask for your understanding. Please know that these imperfections don't diminish the love and effort poured into this book.

As you read and practice with this guide, I hope you'll feel the encouragement and belief I have in you. Chair yoga is more than an exercise—it's a gift you give yourself. It's a chance to honor your body, embrace your breath, and take a moment for the incredible person you are.

If this book inspires even one of you to move a little more freely, smile a little more often, or find a little more peace in your day, then it's been worth every moment of writing.

So, grab a chair, take a deep breath, and let's begin this journey together. Know that I'm cheering for you every step of the way.

With gratitude and warmth,

Tessa Linden

Introduction

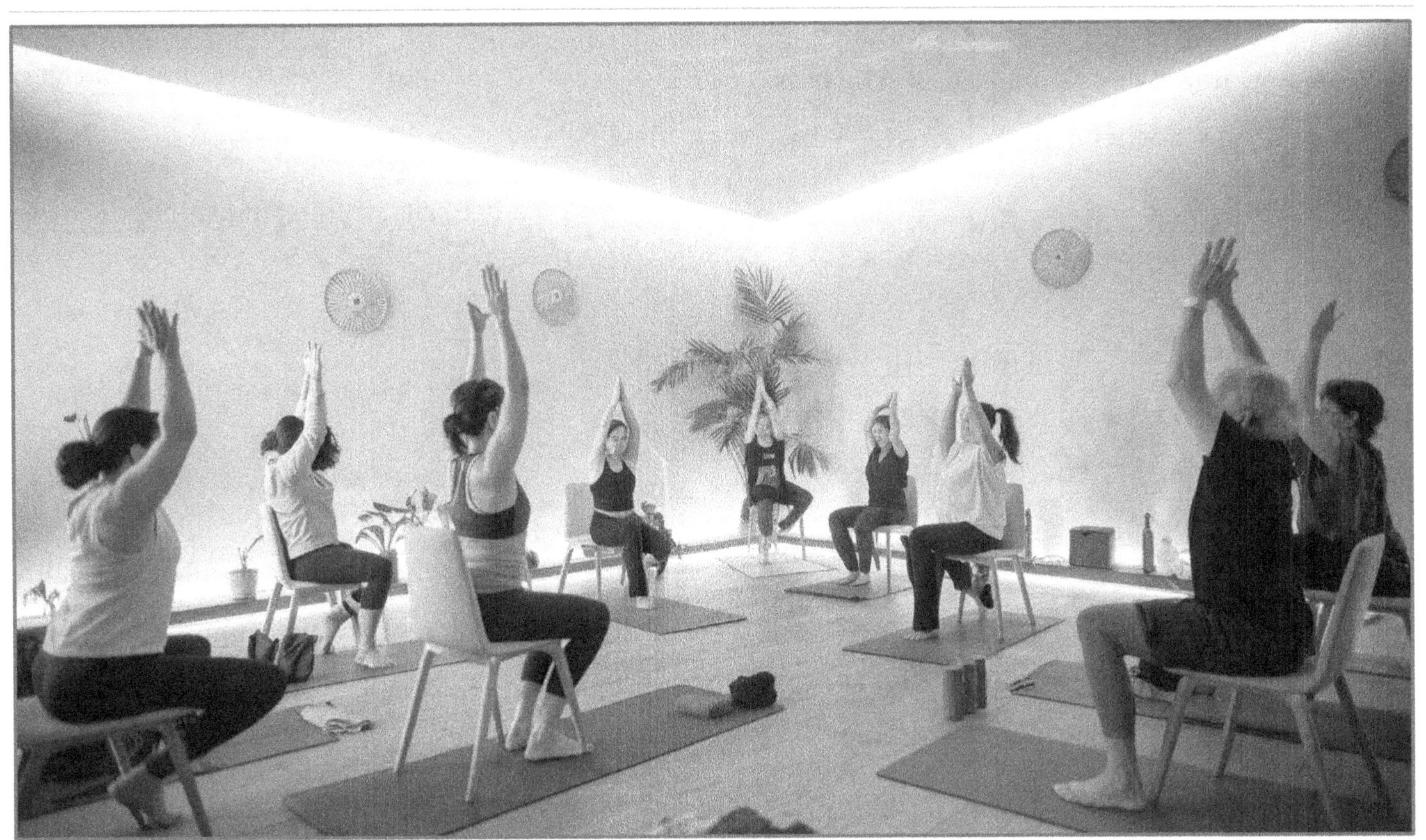

Why Chair Yoga?

Imagine feeling more flexible, energized, and centered—all without leaving your chair. Chair yoga offers a gentle yet powerful way to improve your overall health and well-being, especially for seniors and beginners who may feel daunted by traditional exercise routines.

Chair yoga is not just a workout; it's a lifestyle upgrade. It's a way to strengthen your body, calm your mind, and improve your mobility without the stress of getting on the floor or performing complicated poses. Whether you're looking to regain flexibility, reduce stress, or simply move more in your daily life, chair yoga is an excellent place to start.

Here's why chair yoga is a game-changer:

Accessible for Everyone:

Whether you're new to yoga, recovering from an injury, or managing limited mobility, chair yoga meets you where you are. All you need is a sturdy chair and a few minutes a day to get started.

Improves Mobility and Flexibility:

The gentle stretches and movements help loosen stiff joints, increase your range of motion, and improve posture—all of which are vital for staying independent and active.

Reduces Stress and Boosts Mental Clarity:

Chair yoga combines movement with mindful breathing, reducing tension and calming your mind. It's a simple yet effective way to combat stress and improve focus.

Supports Healthy Aging:

As we age, maintaining strength and balance becomes crucial. Chair yoga strengthens muscles, improves circulation, and helps prevent falls, making it a great ally for healthy aging.

Easy to Fit into a Busy Day:

A 15-minute practice can fit into anyone's schedule. It's quick enough to do during a break, after waking up, or before bedtime, yet effective enough to make a noticeable difference.

A Gateway to a Healthier Lifestyle:

Chair yoga often serves as a stepping stone to more physical activity, better nutrition, and a more mindful approach to life.

No matter your starting point, chair yoga is about progress, not perfection. This guide will be your supportive companion, helping you take small but meaningful steps toward a healthier, happier you.

Are you ready to sit, stretch, and shine? Let's get started!

Benefits of Gentle Exercise for Seniors and Beginners

Gentle exercise, like chair yoga, offers a wealth of benefits tailored to the unique needs of seniors and those just starting their fitness journey. It's more than just physical movement—it's about improving your quality of life in a way that feels manageable and rewarding. Let's explore how gentle exercise can make a real difference for you:

1. Improves Joint Flexibility and Mobility

Stiff joints can limit your movements and affect your daily life. Chair yoga incorporates slow, deliberate stretches that help loosen tight muscles and increase your range of motion. With regular practice, you'll find it easier to bend, twist, and reach comfortably.

2. Builds Strength and Stability

Maintaining muscle strength is key to staying active and independent as you age. Gentle exercises strengthen key muscle groups, especially in your core, arms, and legs. This helps improve balance, which reduces the risk of falls—a major concern for seniors.

3. Boosts Circulation and Heart Health

When you move, your blood flows more freely, delivering oxygen and nutrients throughout your body. Even low-impact activities like chair yoga can improve circulation, support cardiovascular health, and help regulate blood pressure.

4. Supports Mental Well-Being

Gentle exercise isn't just for the body—it's also for the mind. Moving with mindfulness reduces stress and anxiety, while the focus on breathing fosters a sense of calm and clarity. For beginners, this can be a great introduction to the mental benefits of movement.

5. Encourages Healthy Weight Management

Staying active, even at a gentle pace, helps burn calories and improve metabolism. Combined with mindful eating, gentle exercises can support your weight management goals without the intensity of high-impact workouts.

6. Reduces Aches and Pains

If you're dealing with chronic pain, arthritis, or muscle tension, gentle movements can be a soothing remedy. Chair yoga's targeted stretches and poses are designed to ease discomfort while avoiding strain.

7. Boosts Energy and Vitality

Feeling sluggish? A short chair yoga session can energize you by stimulating your body and refreshing your mind. Gentle exercise helps combat fatigue, leaving you more alert and focused throughout the day.

8. Fosters a Sense of Accomplishment

Starting an exercise routine can feel overwhelming, but chair yoga's simplicity makes it approachable. Each time you complete a session, you'll feel a sense of pride in taking a step toward better health.

9. Adaptable to Your Needs

One of the best things about gentle exercise is how adaptable it is. Chair yoga offers modifications for all fitness levels and physical abilities, making it a welcoming practice for everyone, no matter where they're starting from.

A Gentle Start to Big Changes

Remember, it's not about doing more or pushing harder—it's about starting where you are and moving in a way that feels good. Gentle exercise is a sustainable, enjoyable path to better health, and every small step adds up to a brighter, more active future.

Let's keep moving forward—one stretch, one breath, and one smile at a time!

Combining Movement, Mindfulness, and Diet for Success

Achieving overall well-being doesn't come from just one aspect of a healthy lifestyle—it's a balance of movement, mindfulness, and diet. Chair yoga beautifully blends these elements, making it a powerful tool for seniors and beginners who want to feel better, live healthier, and move through life with more ease. Here's how combining these three pillars can create lasting success:

1. Movement: Building Strength and Flexibility

Movement is essential for keeping your body strong and your joints mobile. Chair yoga offers a low-impact way to engage your muscles, improve posture, and boost circulation—all without putting unnecessary strain on your body.

Why it matters: Regular movement helps reduce stiffness, build endurance, and keep your body functioning optimally. Even 15 minutes a day can have profound benefits.

Your goal: Make movement a non-negotiable part of your routine. Think of it as a gift to your body—a way to honor what it can do, no matter your starting point.

2. Mindfulness: Cultivating Inner Peace

Mindfulness is the practice of being present in the moment, and chair yoga makes it easy to integrate this into your day. By focusing on your breath and gentle movements, you create a sense of calm that radiates throughout your life.

Why it matters: Stress and anxiety can affect your physical health as much as inactivity. Practicing mindfulness during chair yoga helps quiet your mind and improve your mental clarity.

Your goal: Approach each yoga session with intention. Use it as an opportunity to tune in to your body, let go of worries, and reconnect with yourself.

3. Diet: Fueling Your Body for Better Results

Movement and mindfulness are powerful, but your body also needs the right fuel to perform at its best. A balanced diet rich in whole foods, lean proteins, healthy fats, and colorful fruits and vegetables provides the energy you need to stay active and focused.

Why it matters: Proper nutrition supports muscle recovery, maintains energy levels, and complements the physical benefits of chair yoga. It's a way to nourish your body inside and out.

Your goal: Pair your chair yoga practice with mindful eating habits. Listen to your body's hunger cues, stay hydrated, and focus on foods that make you feel energized and vibrant.

Creating Your Wellness Trio

Think of movement, mindfulness, and diet as three interconnected parts of a whole. When you combine them, you'll:

Feel more energized to tackle each day.

Manage stress more effectively.

See greater improvements in flexibility, strength, and overall health.

Practical Tips for Success

Start small: Begin with your daily 15-minute chair yoga practice. Add mindfulness by focusing on your breath during poses, and make one healthy change to your meals each week.

Stay consistent: Commit to these habits daily, even if some days are less than perfect. Consistency beats perfection every time.

Celebrate progress: Whether it's touching your toes, feeling calmer, or choosing a healthy snack, every win counts.

A Holistic Path to Health

When you bring movement, mindfulness, and diet together, you create a foundation for a healthier, happier life. Chair yoga is the perfect way to integrate these three elements—gently, effectively, and joyfully.

Your journey doesn't have to be perfect; it just has to begin. Let's take that step together!

Choosing the Right Chair and Setting Up Your Space

Starting your chair yoga journey begins with two simple steps: finding the right chair and creating a space that sets the stage for a calm, focused practice. With these basics in place, you'll feel comfortable, safe, and ready to move.

Choosing the Right Chair

Your chair is the foundation of your practice, so picking the right one is essential. Here's what to look for:

Sturdy and Stable:

Select a chair with a solid frame that won't wobble or tip during your movements. Avoid chairs with wheels or swivel bases. Stability ensures your safety as you stretch and pose.

Supportive Seat:

A firm, flat seat without excessive cushioning is ideal. It provides the support you need while allowing you to sit upright comfortably.

No Armrests (Optional):

While armrests can be helpful for certain modifications, they may restrict your range of motion for some poses. If possible, use a chair without armrests to allow full freedom of movement.

Height Matters:

Choose a chair that lets your feet rest flat on the ground with your knees bent at a 90-degree angle. If your chair is too high, use a footrest; if it's too low, add a cushion to the seat.

Non-Slip Feet:

Ensure the chair has non-slip feet or place it on a non-slip surface to prevent it from sliding as you move.

Setting Up Your Space

Creating a welcoming space for your practice can make all the difference. Here's how to set the stage:

Pick a Quiet Spot:

Find a location free from distractions, noise, or clutter. A calm environment helps you focus on your movements and breathing.

Ample Room to Move:

Ensure you have enough space around your chair to stretch your arms and legs comfortably. Move furniture or items out of the way if necessary.

Add a Yoga Mat or Rug:

Place your chair on a non-slip surface like a

yoga mat or rug. This adds stability and a touch of comfort, especially for foot or hand exercises.

Lighting and Ambiance:

Soft, natural light or gentle indoor lighting creates a relaxing atmosphere. Consider adding a plant or a soothing candle (placed safely) for an inviting touch.

Keep Essentials Nearby:

Have a water bottle, towel, or any yoga props (like blocks or a strap) within arm's reach. This keeps you prepared and focused during your session.

Comfortable Clothing:

Wear loose, breathable clothes that allow you to move freely. Avoid tight or restrictive garments.

Making Your Space Your Own

Your chair yoga practice is a time to focus on yourself, so personalize your space in ways that bring you joy. Maybe it's adding your favorite playlist, practicing near a window with a beautiful view, or including a few moments of quiet reflection before you start.

Safety Tips and Common Modifications

Chair yoga is designed to be gentle and accessible, but prioritizing safety ensures that your practice is both effective and enjoyable. Whether you're a beginner or managing specific health concerns, following these tips and using modifications can help you practice with confidence.

Safety Tips for Chair Yoga

Listen to Your Body

Respect your limits. If a movement feels uncomfortable or causes pain, stop immediately. It's normal to feel a gentle stretch, but you should never feel sharp or intense pain.

Start Slow and Steady

Begin with smaller movements and shorter sessions. As your flexibility and strength improve, gradually increase the intensity and duration of your practice.

Use a Stable Chair

Ensure your chair is sturdy and placed on a non-slip surface. Avoid chairs with wheels or ones that feel unsteady.

Maintain Proper Posture

Sit up straight with your feet flat on the floor, knees at a 90-degree angle. This alignment supports your spine and prevents unnecessary strain.

Avoid Overstretching

It's tempting to push for deeper stretches, but overdoing it can lead to injury. Ease into each pose and stop when you feel a comfortable stretch.

Breathe Consistently

Never hold your breath. Breathe deeply and steadily through your movements, as proper breathing enhances relaxation and oxygen flow.

Consult Your Healthcare Provider

If you have existing health conditions, injuries, or concerns, check with your doctor before starting chair yoga. They can help determine any precautions you should take.

Common Modifications for Chair Yoga

Chair yoga is adaptable to suit your needs, no matter your fitness level or physical limitations. Here are some simple modifications to make poses accessible and comfortable:

Limited Flexibility in the Hips or Legs

Modification: Use a rolled-up towel or small cushion under your thighs for added support. Adjust your foot placement to find a comfortable position.

Difficulty Reaching Arms Overhead

Modification: Reach only as far as feels comfortable or keep your hands on your thighs while visualizing the stretch. You can also clasp your hands in front of your chest instead.

Balance Concerns

Modification: Hold onto the sides of the chair or place your hands on your lap for stability during poses that involve twisting or leaning.

Limited Neck Mobility

Modification: Keep your neck in a neutral position and avoid poses that require looking up or down excessively. Focus on gentle shoulder movements instead.

Trouble Maintaining Posture

Modification: Place a small cushion or folded towel at the small of your back for additional lumbar support.

Sensitive Knees or Joints

Modification: Keep movements smaller and avoid poses that require deep bending. Use a softer chair cushion if needed.

Difficulty Standing (if part of your routine involves standing poses)

Modification: Perform standing poses seated by mimicking the movement. For example, a seated Warrior Pose can be done by extending one leg forward and reaching your arms upward.

Tips for People with Limited Mobility

Focus on Upper Body Movements:

If standing or moving your lower body is difficult, prioritize poses that involve the arms, shoulders, neck, and upper back. For example, seated shoulder rolls or arm stretches can build strength and improve flexibility.

Engage Through Visualization:

For movements that are physically challenging, try visualizing the motion. Studies show that imagining movement can stimulate the muscles and improve neural pathways.

Keep Sessions Shorter:

Begin with 5-10 minutes of practice, gradually increasing duration as you build strength and confidence.

Use Props for Support:

Place a rolled towel or cushion behind your lower back for lumbar support. Resistance bands can help with stretches that are hard to reach.

Suggestions for Those Practicing in Smaller Spaces

Prioritize a Clear Area Around the Chair:

Even in small spaces, ensure there's at least a 2-foot radius around your chair for safe arm and leg movements.

Use Compact Props:

Choose smaller yoga aids like resistance bands, small weights, or a folded towel instead of bulky equipment.

Opt for Multi-Use Spaces:

Your practice space doesn't have to be permanent. A dining chair in your living room or bedroom corner can serve as a temporary yoga spot.

Make Use of Vertical Space:

Practice near a wall for support during standing or balance-based movements, doubling your safety in a small area.

Keep it Simple:

Focus on poses that don't require large arm or leg extensions. Seated spinal twists, gentle side bends, or neck stretches are perfect for tight spaces.

Advice for Adapting Chair Yoga for Taller or Shorter Individuals

Adjust Chair Height:

Taller individuals may need a cushion to raise the seat height for optimal knee alignment, while shorter individuals can use a footrest to ensure their feet are flat on the ground.

Modify Arm Movements:

For taller individuals, ensure arms don't overextend by slightly bending elbows during overhead stretches. Shorter practitioners can bring their hands only as high as comfortable.

Customize Leg Stretches:

Taller individuals may need more space for leg extensions; ensure nothing obstructs the area in front of the chair. Shorter individuals can place blocks or books under their feet during certain stretches for better support.

Adjust the Chair Position:

Position the chair closer to a wall or support structure if taller practitioners feel unsteady during stretching.

General Tips for a Safer Practice

Warm Up First: Gentle stretches and movements prepare your body for deeper poses, reducing the risk of strain.

Use Props if Needed: Yoga straps, resistance bands, or even a scarf can assist with stretches. Yoga blocks or books can provide extra support for your feet or hands.

Stay Hydrated: Keep a water bottle nearby to stay refreshed, especially during longer sessions.

End with Relaxation: Finish each session with deep breathing or a simple seated meditation to reset and relax your body.

Chair Yoga, Your Way

Safety and comfort are key to a sustainable chair yoga practice. Remember, there's no rush to master every pose—what matters most is that you feel supported and confident as you move. Adjust as needed, and enjoy the journey at your own pace.

What to Expect from a 15-Minute Daily Practice

A 15-minute chair yoga session may seem brief, but it can be surprisingly effective when done consistently. Over time, you'll begin to notice improvements in flexibility, strength, balance, and mental clarity. Here's what you can expect from your daily practice and how to get the most out of it:

Immediate Benefits:

Increased Energy

Starting your day with chair yoga can help wake up your body and mind. The gentle movements stimulate circulation, helping you feel more alert and energized.

Improved Focus

As you move through poses, you'll practice being present, which enhances your mental clarity. The simple act of focusing on your breath and body can improve concentration.

Stress Relief

The deep breathing and mindfulness practiced in chair yoga can help reduce stress and anxiety, leaving you feeling calmer and more centered.

Relief from Tension

Even in just 15 minutes, chair yoga can target common tension points in the body, like your shoulders, neck, and back. By stretching these areas, you'll feel a greater sense of physical ease.

Long-Term Benefits:

Improved Flexibility

With regular practice, you'll notice an increase in joint mobility and flexibility. Poses that once felt stiff or challenging will become easier over time.

Stronger Muscles

Even though chair yoga is low-impact, it still helps strengthen muscles, particularly in your core, arms, and legs. This added strength supports your posture and daily activities.

Better Balance and Coordination

Chair yoga includes movements that engage your balance and coordination, which improves over time, reducing the risk of falls and improving stability.

Pain Management

Many people find that regular chair yoga helps alleviate chronic pain, especially in areas like the hips, knees, and lower back. The gentle stretching and strengthening of muscles can provide relief from stiffness and discomfort.

How It Feels During Practice:

Gentle Movement

Chair yoga is designed to be accessible, so you'll feel supported in every pose. The movements are slow and controlled, allowing you to ease into each stretch at your own pace.

Increased Body Awareness

As you move through poses, you'll become more aware of how your body feels. This awareness helps you better understand your body's needs and limitations, and it guides you to make modifications when necessary.

Breathing Awareness

Focusing on your breath is a key aspect of chair yoga. As you practice deep, steady breathing, you'll feel more connected to your body and less distracted by outside thoughts.

A Sense of Calm

Towards the end of each session, especially if you finish with relaxation or breathing exercises, you'll feel a sense of calm and relaxation, which helps set a positive tone for the rest of your day.

Tips for Maximizing Your 15-Minute Practice:

Be Consistent

While 15 minutes may seem like a small commitment, consistency is key. Practicing every day, or as often as possible, ensures you see the best results.

Focus on Quality, Not Quantity

It's not about rushing through each pose; it's about being present and moving with intention. Focus on quality rather than trying to fit as many poses as possible into your short session.

Integrate Breathing and Mindfulness

Don't just stretch—breathe. The power of chair yoga lies in combining gentle movement with mindful breathing. Incorporating this balance into your routine will enhance your results.

Modify as Needed

If something doesn't feel right, modify the pose or skip it. Chair yoga should never feel painful. Use props or adjust your range of motion to suit your comfort level.

Track Your Progress

Keep a journal or use a progress tracker to note how you feel after each session. Over time, you'll see improvements that motivate you to keep going.

What to Expect Over Time:

More Flexibility in Your Body

As you consistently practice, your body will gradually become more flexible. This means you'll be able to reach further, stretch deeper, and hold poses with ease.

Improved Strength and Tone

The muscles you engage during chair yoga will strengthen, especially in your core, arms, and legs. You'll begin to notice more muscle tone and strength with regular practice.

Better Mobility and Posture

With a daily practice, you'll find that your posture improves, and daily movements (like standing, sitting, or walking) become easier and more fluid.

Less Stress and More Relaxation

As your body becomes more relaxed, your mind follows suit. You'll experience a greater sense of calm, reduced anxiety, and an improved ability to cope with stress.

The Takeaway

Starting with just 15 minutes a day can lead to profound physical and mental changes. Chair yoga is a simple yet powerful tool for enhancing your flexibility, strength, and peace of mind. Whether you practice in the morning to energize, in the middle of the day to relieve tension, or at night to wind down, your daily routine will provide lasting benefits for your body and mind.

Common Mistakes to Avoid in Chair Yoga

While chair yoga is a gentle and accessible practice, it's still important to approach it mindfully. Avoiding these common mistakes will help you get the most out of your practice and ensure that it's both safe and effective for your body.

1. Overstretching or Pushing Beyond Comfort

Mistake: Trying to stretch too far or too fast in an effort to see quick results.

Why It's a Mistake: Overstretching can lead to strain or injury, especially for seniors or beginners with less flexibility.

Solution: Always listen to your body. Stretch to the point of mild tension, not pain. It's okay to hold back a little—yoga is about gradual improvement, not forcing your body.

2. Not Using Proper Alignment

Mistake: Practicing yoga with poor posture or slumping in the chair, which can strain your back, neck, or shoulders.

Why It's a Mistake: Incorrect alignment can cause discomfort and lead to chronic pain, especially when done repeatedly over time.

Solution: Sit with your feet flat on the floor, knees at a 90-degree angle, and your spine tall and elongated. Avoid rounding your back or dropping your shoulders forward. Focus on maintaining good posture throughout each pose.

3. Skipping the Warm-Up or Cool-Down

Mistake: Jumping straight into challenging poses or finishing abruptly without cooling down.

Why It's a Mistake: Warm-ups prepare your muscles for movement, and cool-downs allow your body to relax after exercise. Skipping these steps can increase your risk of injury or leave you feeling tight and tense.

Solution: Begin with gentle stretches like

shoulder rolls or neck stretches to warm up your body. End each session with slow, calming stretches and deep breathing to release any tension built up during the practice.

4. Holding Your Breath

Mistake: Forgetting to breathe while holding poses or trying to "hold" your breath during challenging stretches.

Why It's a Mistake: Breath is essential in yoga—it helps you stay relaxed, supports muscle engagement, and allows your body to release tension.

Solution: Focus on deep, consistent breathing throughout your practice. Inhale through your nose and exhale through your mouth, coordinating your breath with your movements. If you feel tight or tense, take a moment to reset your breath.

5. Practicing with Poor Chair Support

Mistake: Using a chair that's unstable, too low, or too high, which can lead to discomfort or injury.

Why It's a Mistake: An improper chair can disrupt your alignment and balance, making poses harder to execute safely.

Solution: Choose a sturdy chair with a firm seat, and make sure your feet can touch the ground comfortably. Your knees should be at a 90-degree angle when seated, and your back should be fully supported. A chair without armrests is ideal, but if yours has them, make sure they don't get in the way of your movements.

6. Not Modifying Poses for Your Body's Needs

Mistake: Doing poses exactly as shown, even if they don't feel comfortable or accessible for your body.

Why It's a Mistake: Not all poses are suitable for everyone, especially if you have mobility restrictions, arthritis, or other physical limitations.

Solution: Chair yoga is all about modification! If a pose feels too intense or doesn't work for you, modify it. Use props like cushions, blocks, or resistance bands to support your movements. Don't hesitate to reduce the range of motion or skip poses that don't feel right.

7. Ignoring Pain or Discomfort

Mistake: Continuing a pose or movement even when it causes pain or discomfort.

Why It's a Mistake: Pain is a clear signal from your body that something isn't right. Ignoring pain can lead to injury and setbacks in your practice.

Solution: Always listen to your body. If a pose is causing pain, stop immediately, adjust the posture, or switch to a different exercise. It's important to practice yoga safely, with mindfulness.

8. Rushing Through Poses

Mistake: Moving too quickly from one pose to the next in an attempt to complete the routine faster.

Why It's a Mistake: Yoga is about quality, not speed. Rushing through poses can prevent you from getting the full benefit of each movement and increase the risk of injury.

Solution: Slow down and give yourself time to fully experience each pose. Focus on alignment, breathing, and mindful movement. Stay in each pose for a few breaths to really engage your muscles and stretch.

9. Not Staying Consistent

Mistake: Practicing chair yoga sporadically or only when you feel like it, rather than making it part of a daily routine.

Why It's a Mistake: Consistency is key to seeing lasting results in flexibility, strength, and overall health. Skipping days can hinder progress and make it harder to maintain the habit.

Solution: Set aside a consistent time each day to practice. Even 15 minutes a day can lead to significant improvements in your physical and mental well-being. Make it a daily ritual to help build and maintain the habit.

10. Comparing Yourself to Others

Mistake: Comparing your progress to others or feeling frustrated when you don't see instant results.

Why It's a Mistake: Yoga is a personal practice, and everyone's body is different. Comparing yourself to others can lead to disappointment and discouragement.

Solution: Focus on your own journey. Celebrate the small wins and progress you make, and remember that yoga is about listening to your body, not competing with others.

The Takeaway

Avoiding these common mistakes will help you maintain a safe, effective, and enjoyable chair yoga practice. Remember, chair yoga is not about perfection—it's about progress, connection, and self-care. Always listen to your body, be patient with yourself, and most importantly, enjoy the process.

The Power of 15 Minutes: Why Short, Consistent Practice is Effective

Life can feel overwhelming, especially when it comes to finding time for exercise. However, chair yoga doesn't demand hours of your day to make a meaningful impact. By committing just 15 minutes daily, you can reap significant benefits for your body, mind, and overall well-being. Here's why short, consistent practice works so effectively:

1. It's Easy to Commit To

Why It Works: A short session fits seamlessly into even the busiest of schedules. Whether you're starting your day, taking a midday break, or unwinding in the evening, finding 15 minutes is manageable for almost everyone.

The Impact: When something feels achievable, you're more likely to stick with it. Over time, this consistency builds habits that lead to lasting results.

2. Builds Momentum for Bigger Goals

Why It Works: Starting with just 15 minutes creates a sense of accomplishment, which motivates you to continue. This small daily win can lead to more ambitious health and fitness goals as you gain confidence in your abilities.

The Impact: Once chair yoga becomes part of your routine, you may naturally start exploring longer or more varied sessions, or even complementing your practice with other wellness activities.

3. Promotes Physical Health Without Overwhelming Your Body

Why It Works: Short sessions of chair yoga provide gentle, low-impact movement that improves flexibility, strength, and circulation without exhausting you. For seniors and beginners, this balance is essential for staying energized and avoiding fatigue.

The Impact: Over time, these consistent, small efforts compound, leading to noticeable improvements in joint mobility, posture, and overall strength.

4. Enhances Mental Focus and Reduces Stress

Why It Works: A brief yoga session gives you a dedicated moment to pause, breathe, and reset. Practicing mindfulness for even 15 minutes helps reduce stress, improve focus, and boost your mood.

The Impact: Regular relaxation practices improve mental clarity and emotional resilience, helping you handle daily challenges with a calmer, more balanced outlook.

5. Encourages Long-Term Habit Formation

Why It Works: A short time commitment removes the intimidation factor often associated with starting a new routine. By keeping it simple, you'll find it easier to establish yoga as a non-negotiable part of your day.

The Impact: Once the habit is ingrained, it becomes second nature, just like brushing your teeth. This consistency is the secret to long-term wellness.

6. Delivers Cumulative Benefits Over Time

Why It Works: While 15 minutes may feel modest, the effects of daily practice add up. You'll notice increased flexibility, improved posture, and better energy levels as the days and weeks go by.

The Impact: The cumulative benefits of regular chair yoga can rival those of longer, more strenuous workout routines, especially for those who are new to exercise or have mobility limitations.

7. Reduces the Risk of Injury

Why It Works: A shorter session keeps your body moving without overloading your joints or muscles, reducing the likelihood of strain or injury.

The Impact: By gradually building strength and flexibility, you'll support your body's ability to perform daily activities safely and confidently.

Making It Happen: A Few Practical Tips

Consistency Is Key: Aim to practice at the same time each day to make it a habit.

Start Slow: If 15 minutes feels like too much initially, begin with 5-10 minutes and gradually increase.

Stay Flexible: You can always adapt your session to fit your energy level and needs for the day.

The Takeaway

Fifteen minutes may seem small, but it's enough to unlock big changes in your health and well-being. By making this simple, consistent commitment to chair yoga, you're investing in a practice that nurtures your body, clears your mind, and strengthens your spirit. Small steps lead to big results—your 15 minutes today is the foundation for a healthier, happier tomorrow.

Seated Shoulder Rolls

Seated shoulder rolls are a simple and effective warm-up exercise to release tension, improve posture, and increase mobility in the shoulders and upper back.

What You Need

- A sturdy, stable chair without wheels.
- Optional: A cushion for added comfort.

Step-by-Step Instructions

Set Your Position:

- Sit upright on the chair with your feet flat on the floor, hip-width apart.
- Keep your spine straight and shoulders relaxed.
- Rest your hands on your thighs or at your sides.

Lift Your Shoulders:

- Take a deep inhale and slowly lift both shoulders toward your ears.
- Hold this position for a moment, feeling the gentle stretch in your shoulder muscles.

Roll Backward:

- Exhale as you slowly roll your shoulders backward, drawing them down and squeezing your shoulder blades gently together.
- Allow your shoulders to return to their natural resting position.

Repeat the Motion:

- Perform this backward rolling motion 5-10 times in a slow and controlled manner.

Reverse the Direction:

- After completing the backward rolls, reverse the movement. Inhale as you lift your shoulders, exhale as you roll them forward.
- **Repeat for another 5-10 times.**

Common Mistakes to Avoid

- Hunching Forward: Keep your chest open and maintain an upright posture.
- Rushing the Movements: Perform the rolls slowly and smoothly to maximize the stretch.

Benefits

- Loosens tight muscles in the shoulders and neck.
- Improves posture by increasing awareness and mobility.
- Boosts circulation and warms up the upper body.

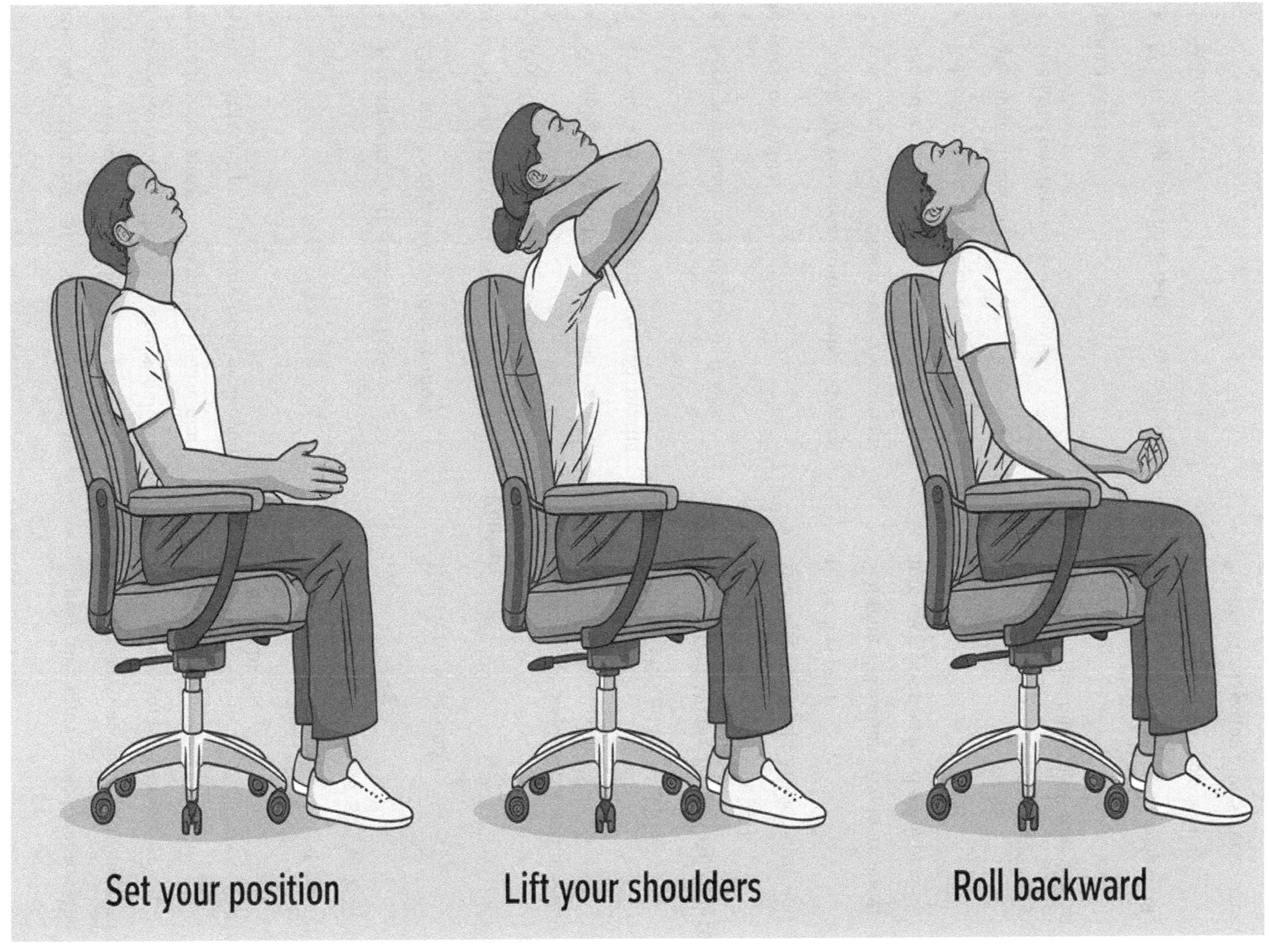

Set your position
Lift your shoulders
Roll backward

Gentle Neck Stretches

Gentle neck stretches are simple movements designed to reduce stiffness, improve flexibility, and relieve tension in the neck and shoulders. They're ideal for anyone looking to release daily stress or counteract poor posture from prolonged sitting.

What You Need

- A sturdy chair with a straight back.
- Optional: A cushion for added comfort.

Step-by-Step Instructions

Get in Position:

- Sit upright with both feet flat on the ground and your back supported by the chair.
- Keep your hands resting on your thighs.

Side Stretch (Right):

- Slowly tilt your head to the right, bringing your right ear closer to your right shoulder.
- Relax your left shoulder down, avoiding any upward tension.
- Hold this position for 5-10 seconds.

Return to Center:

- Slowly bring your head back to an upright position.

Side Stretch (Left):

- Repeat the same movement on the left side, tilting your head to bring your left ear closer to your left shoulder.
- Hold for 5-10 seconds.

Forward Stretch:

- Gently lower your chin toward your chest, feeling a stretch along the back of your neck.
- Hold for 5-10 seconds.

Repeat:

- Perform the sequence 2-3 times, moving slowly and smoothly.

Common Mistakes to Avoid

- Tilting Your Whole Body: Keep your torso still and only move your neck.
- Straining the Neck: Move gently and stop if you feel pain.
- Skipping Relaxation: Avoid rushing; relax into each position for the full benefit.

Benefits

- Reduces neck and shoulder tension.
- Improves flexibility and mobility in the neck area.
- Enhances posture and helps prevent stiffness from prolonged sitting.
- Promotes relaxation and reduces stress.

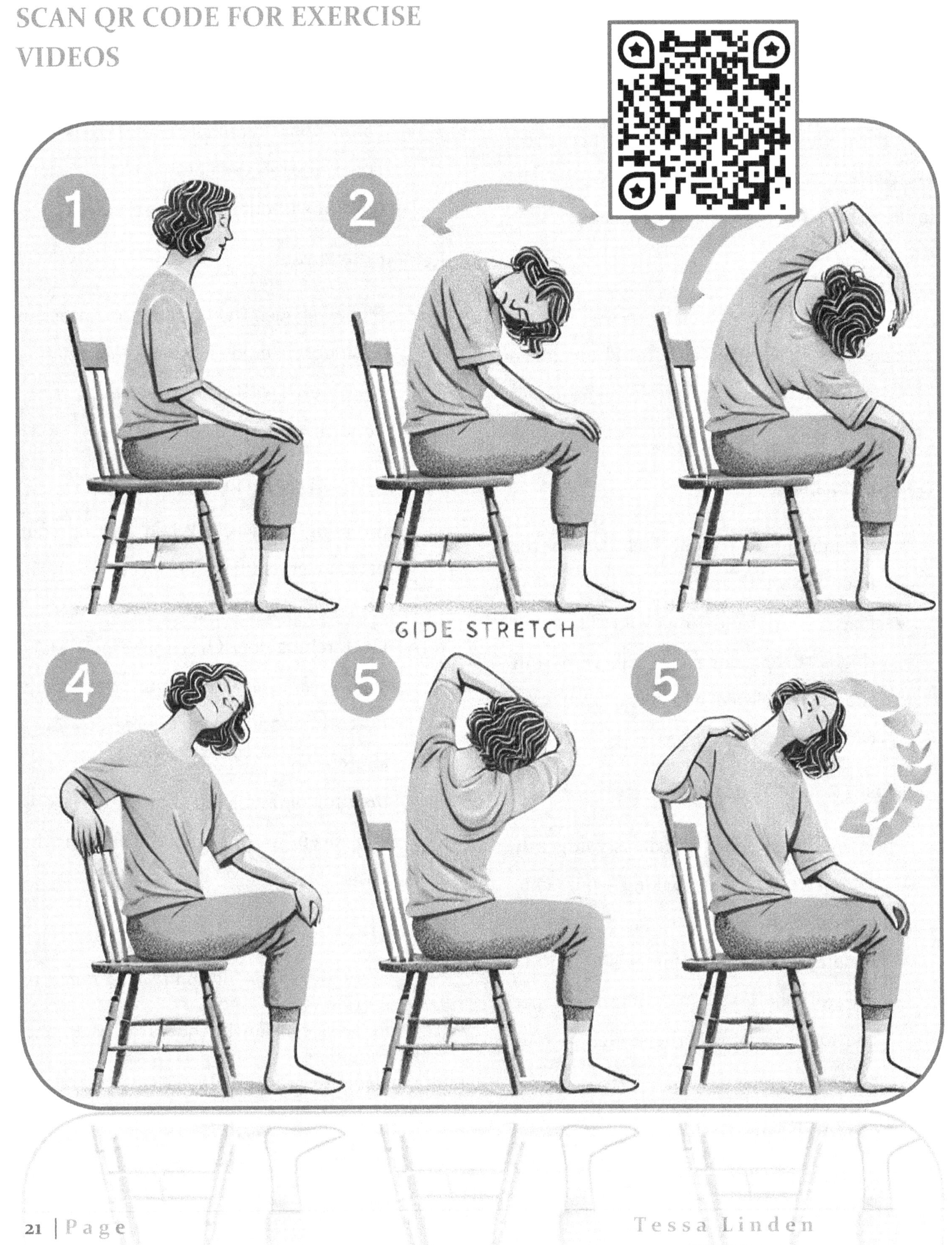
GIDE STRETCH

Seated Cat-Cow Stretch

It combines a forward rounding motion (Cat) and an arching motion (Cow) to increase mobility in the spine, shoulders, and neck. This exercise is ideal for relieving stiffness, especially in the lower back and upper back areas.

What You Need

- A sturdy chair with no armrests.
- Optional: A cushion or towel for added comfort.

Step-by-Step Instructions

Set Your Position:

- Sit upright with your feet flat on the floor, hip-width apart.
- Place your hands on your knees or thighs. Keep your spine tall, with your shoulders relaxed and away from your ears.

Cat Pose (Round Your Back):

- Inhale deeply, then exhale as you gently round your back, tucking your chin toward your chest.
- Imagine drawing your belly button toward your spine, stretching the upper and lower back. Feel the stretch in your spine.

Cow Pose (Arch Your Back):

- Inhale deeply as you arch your back, lifting your chest and chin toward the ceiling.
- Draw your shoulder blades back and down to open the chest, and gently look upward without straining your neck.

Repeat the Flow:

- Move between the Cat and Cow poses in a smooth, fluid motion, coordinating your breath with each movement.
- Perform 5-10 rounds of Cat-Cow.

Common Mistakes to Avoid

- Straining the Neck: When arching your back, avoid craning your neck too much. Keep the movement gentle.
- Overarching or Over-rounding: Make sure you move within your comfortable range of motion. Don't force any deep stretch.
- Breath Holding: Keep your breath steady and deep as you move between the poses.

Benefits

- Increases spinal flexibility and range of motion.
- Relieves tension in the back, neck, and shoulders.
- Helps to reduce stiffness from sitting or poor posture.
- Promotes relaxation through mindful breathing.

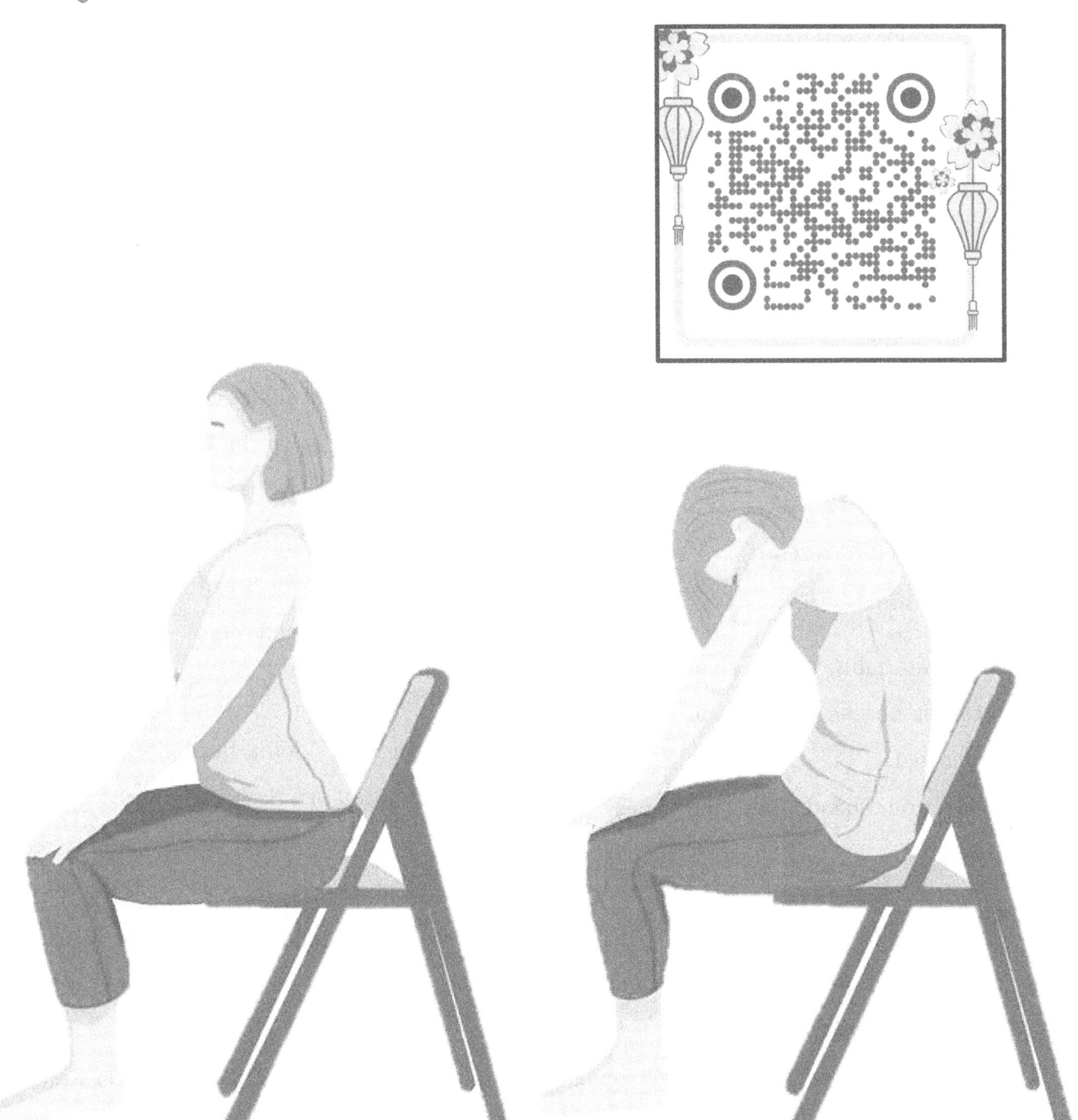

Seated Cat-Cow Stretch

Wrist and Ankle Rotations

Wrist and ankle rotations are simple yet effective exercises to increase joint mobility, reduce stiffness, and promote circulation in the wrists and ankles. These exercises are particularly beneficial for people who spend a lot of time typing, writing, or walking.

What You Need

- A sturdy chair.
- Optional: A cushion or towel for added comfort.

Step-by-Step Instructions

Set Your Position:

- Sit comfortably in the chair with your feet flat on the ground and your back supported.
- Relax your hands on your knees or thighs.

Wrist Rotations:

- Extend your arms in front of you, or place your hands on your thighs.
- Slowly rotate your wrists in a circular motion, making big, smooth circles.
- Perform 5 rotations clockwise and 5 counterclockwise.

Ankle Rotations:

- Lift one foot off the ground and rotate your ankle in a circular motion.
- Perform 5 rotations clockwise and 5 counterclockwise on each foot.
- Repeat for the other foot.

Common Mistakes to Avoid

- Forcing the Movement: Rotate your wrists and ankles gently to avoid strain.
- Not Engaging the Rest of the Body: Keep your posture straight and relaxed as you perform the rotations.
- Holding Your Breath: Breathe deeply and steadily as you rotate.

Benefits

- Increases joint flexibility and range of motion in wrists and ankles.
- Improves circulation and reduces stiffness.
- Helps relieve discomfort caused by repetitive movements or prolonged sitting.
- Promotes relaxation and body awareness.

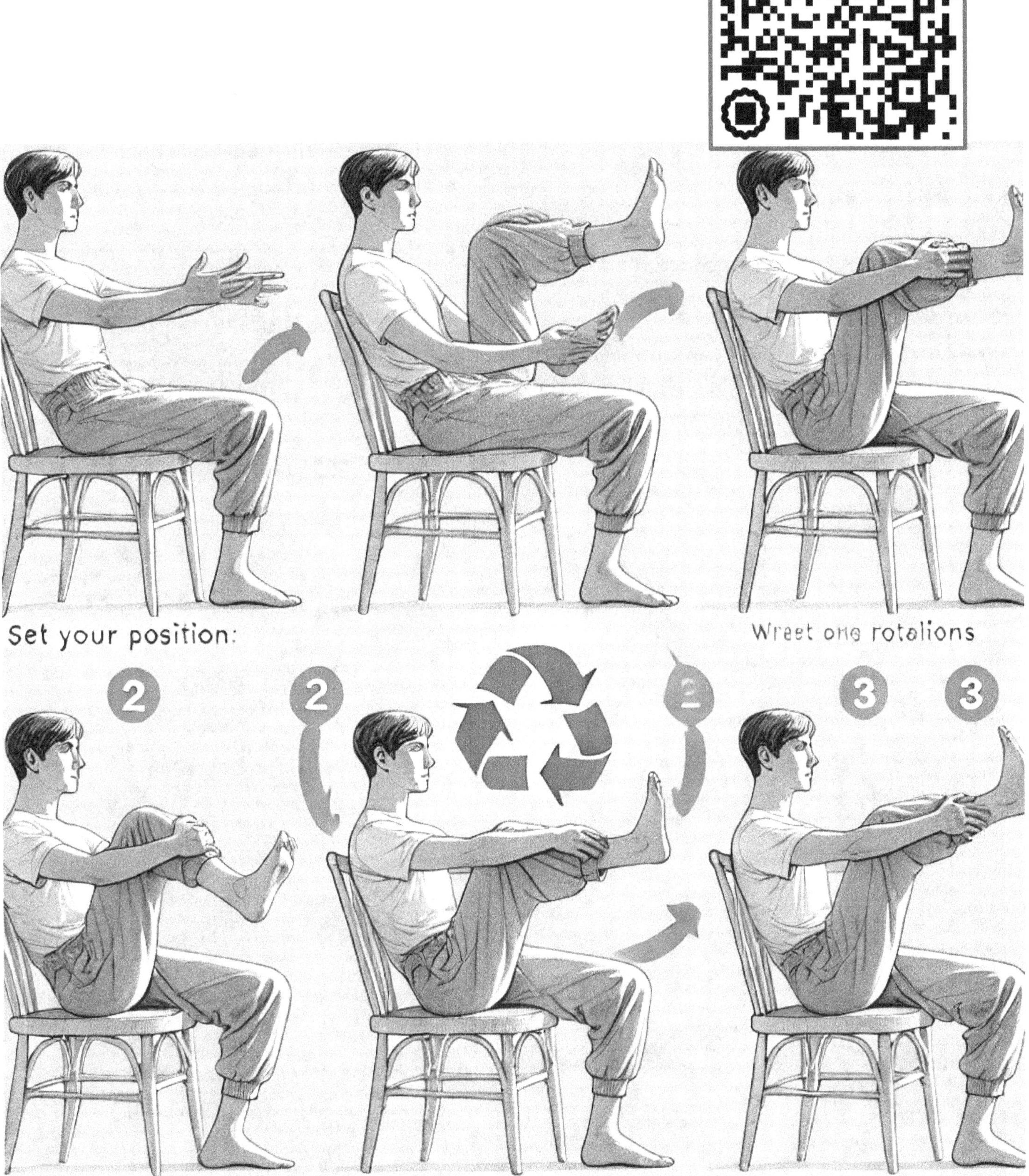
Set your position:
Wreet one rotalions
2
2
2
3
3

Seated Side Stretches

Seated side stretches are a great way to lengthen the muscles on the sides of your body, especially the torso and obliques. These stretches also help improve flexibility and mobility in the spine, making it easier to move and twist. It's a fantastic stretch for those who need to relieve tension in the back, neck, or shoulders.

What You Need

- A sturdy chair.
- Optional: A cushion for added comfort.

Common Mistakes to Avoid

- Leaning Forward or Backward: Keep your body facing forward while performing the stretch to target the side muscles.
- Overstretching: Stretch to a point where you feel a gentle pull, but not pain.
- Holding Your Breath: Remember to breathe deeply throughout the stretch.

Benefits

- Improves flexibility in the sides, back, and shoulders.
- Lengthens the spine and relieves stiffness.
- Promotes better posture by opening the chest and side muscles.
- Reduces tension from daily activities or sitting.

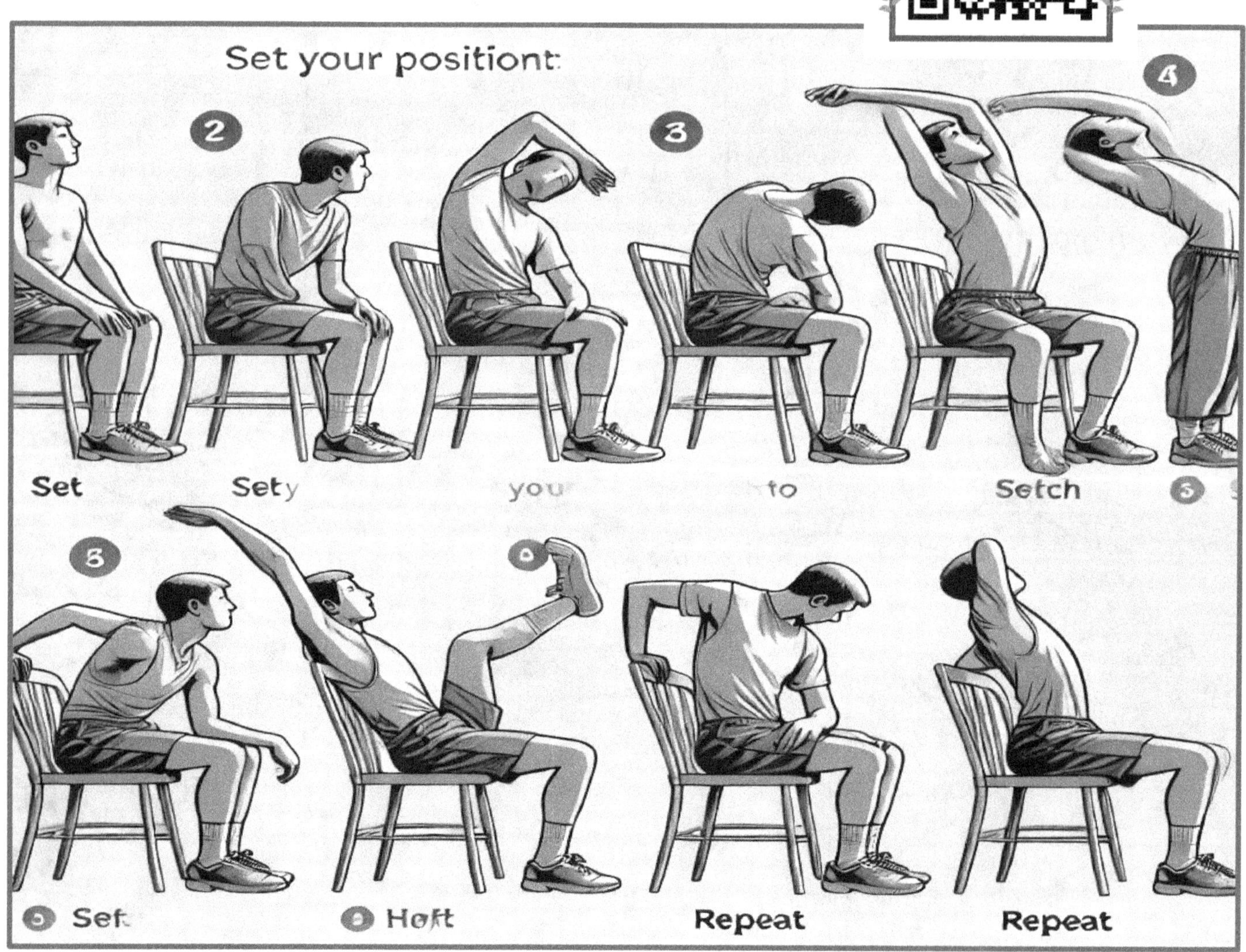

Energizing Morning Routine
Seated Sun Salutation

Seated Sun Salutation is a modified version of the traditional yoga sequence designed for those who prefer or need to practice while seated. This flow engages the entire body, stretches major muscle groups, and incorporates mindful breathing for a calming yet energizing effect.

What You Need

- A sturdy chair without armrests.
- Optional: Comfortable clothing to allow full movement.

Step-by-Step Instructions

Mountain Pose (Seated):

- Sit upright with your feet flat on the floor and your hands resting on your thighs.
- Lengthen your spine, relax your shoulders, and take a deep breath in.

Raise Arms Overhead:

- Inhale deeply and sweep your arms up toward the ceiling, palms facing each other.
- Keep your shoulders relaxed as you lengthen your torso.

Forward Fold (Seated):

- Exhale as you hinge forward at the hips, reaching your hands toward your shins or feet.
- Let your head relax toward your knees, keeping the movement gentle.

Halfway Lift:

- Inhale as you place your hands on your thighs and lift your chest halfway up.
- Keep your back flat and gaze forward slightly.

Seated Backbend:

- Exhale and sit upright, bringing your hands to your lower back or holding the sides of the chair.
- Gently lift your chest and look upward, opening your heart toward the ceiling.

Return to Mountain Pose:

- Inhale and return to the starting position with your hands on your thighs.

Repeat the Flow:

- Perform this flow 3-5 times, moving slowly and mindfully with your breath.

Common Mistakes to Avoid

- Straining the Neck: Avoid overextending your neck during the backbend; keep the movement gentle.
- Rushing the Flow: Move slowly, focusing on your breath to maximize relaxation and benefits.
- Forgetting Alignment: Keep your feet flat and your back straight throughout the sequence.

Benefits

- Stretches the spine, shoulders, and hamstrings.

- Improves flexibility and mobility in the upper and lower body.
- Promotes mindful breathing and relaxation.
- Boosts circulation and energy levels.

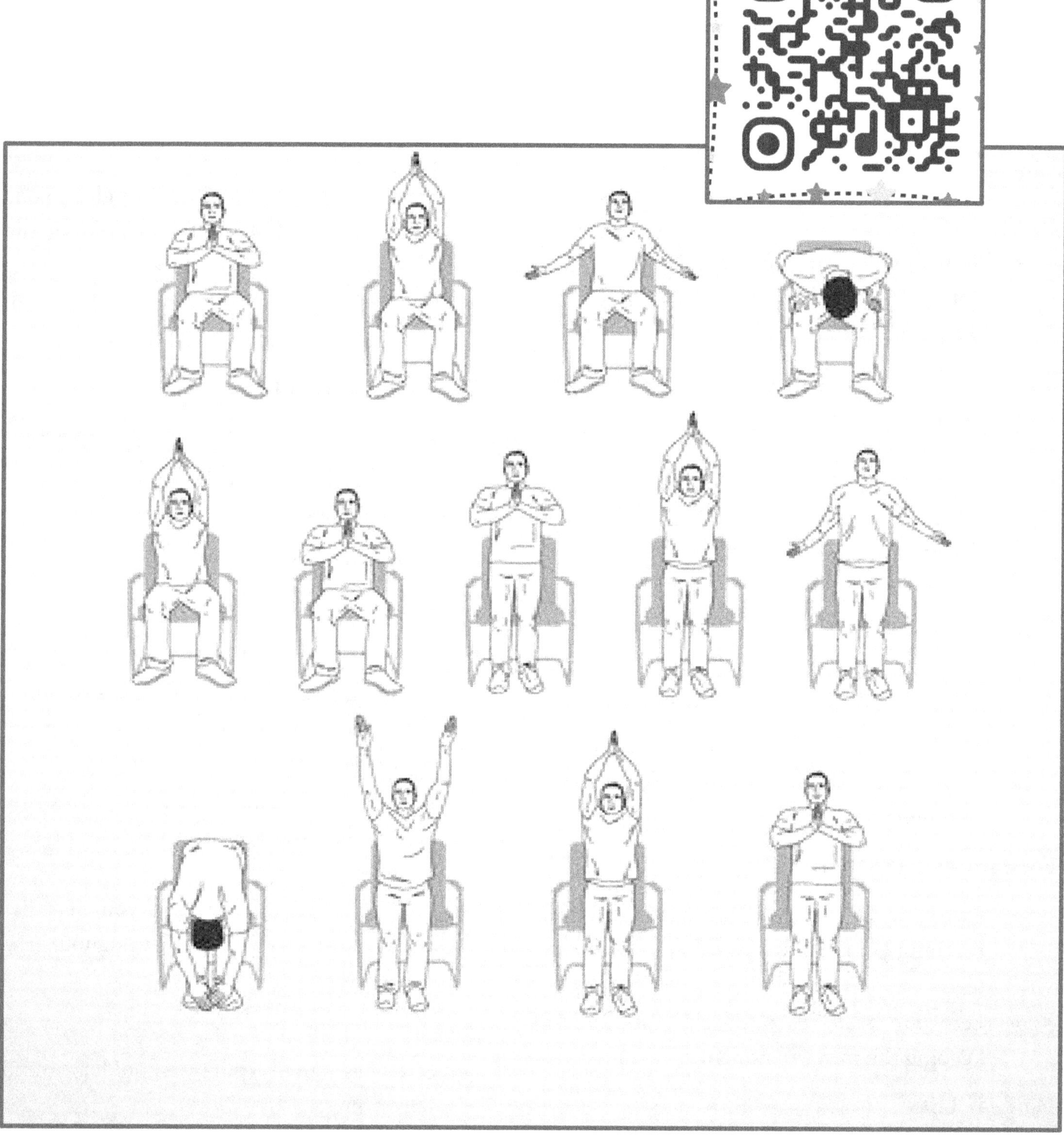

Chair Warrior II is a seated adaptation of the classic yoga pose, designed to strengthen the legs, arms, and core while improving balance and posture. It's perfect for building stability and confidence in movement.

What You Need

- A sturdy chair.
- Optional: Light dumbbells (for extra arm strength, if desired).

Step-by-Step Instructions

Set Your Position:

- Sit on the edge of the chair with your feet flat on the floor, hip-width apart.
- Keep your back straight and your shoulders relaxed.

Extend One Leg:

- Turn your torso slightly to the right and extend your right leg out to the side.
- Your right foot should point outward, and your left knee stays bent at a 90-degree angle.

Raise Your Arms:

- Inhale as you extend your arms out to the sides at shoulder height, palms facing down.
- Keep your arms strong and active, reaching outward.

Hold the Pose:

- Gaze softly over your right hand and maintain the position for 5-10 breaths.
- Engage your core and keep your back tall.

Switch Sides:

- Slowly lower your arms and return to the center.
- Repeat the pose on the left side by extending your left leg and turning your torso to the left.

Common Mistakes to Avoid

- Collapsing the Chest: Keep your chest open and your spine tall throughout the pose.
- Overextending the Arms: Stretch your arms gently; they should feel active but not strained.
- **Lifting the Hips:** Keep both sitting bones grounded on the chair for stability.

Benefits

- Strengthens the legs, arms, and shoulders.
- Improves posture and spinal alignment.
- Enhances balance and stability.
- Boosts confidence and body awareness.

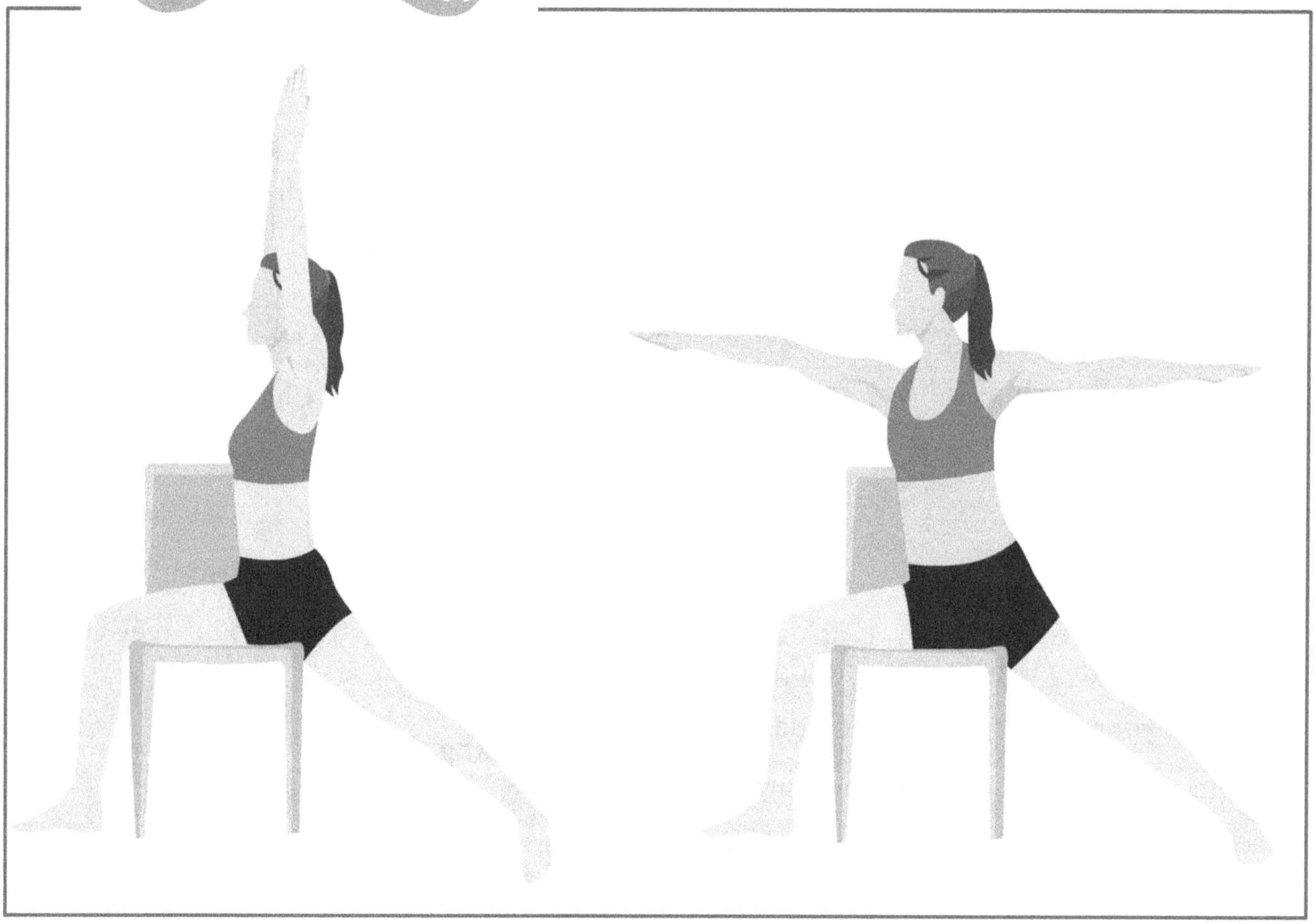

Chair Warrior II

The Seated Spinal Twist is a simple yet effective pose for increasing spinal flexibility and improving digestion. It gently stretches the back and oblique muscles while promoting relaxation and a sense of centeredness.

What You Need

- A sturdy chair without armrests.
- Optional: Cushion or folded towel for added comfort.

Step-by-Step Instructions

Starting Position:

- Sit tall on the chair with your feet flat on the floor, hip-width apart.
- Place your hands on your thighs, and engage your core.

Prepare to Twist:

- Inhale deeply, lengthening your spine as you sit upright.

Twist to One Side:

- Exhale as you gently rotate your torso to the right.
- Place your right hand on the backrest or seat of the chair for support, and your left hand on your right thigh.

Deepen the Stretch:

- Keep your chest open and your gaze over your right shoulder.
- Hold the twist for 3-5 breaths, lengthening the spine with each inhale and deepening the twist slightly with each exhale.

Return to Center:

- Inhale as you slowly unwind and return to the starting position.
- Switch Sides:
- Repeat the twist on your left side, holding for the same duration.

Common Mistakes to Avoid

- Rushing the Movement: Take your time to avoid straining your spine or neck.
- Forcing the Twist: Twist only as far as is comfortable without pain or discomfort.
- Slouching: Keep your back tall and your shoulders relaxed throughout the pose.

Benefits

- Improves spinal mobility and flexibility.
- Aids digestion by gently massaging abdominal organs.
- Relieves tension in the back and shoulders.
- Enhances posture and core strength.

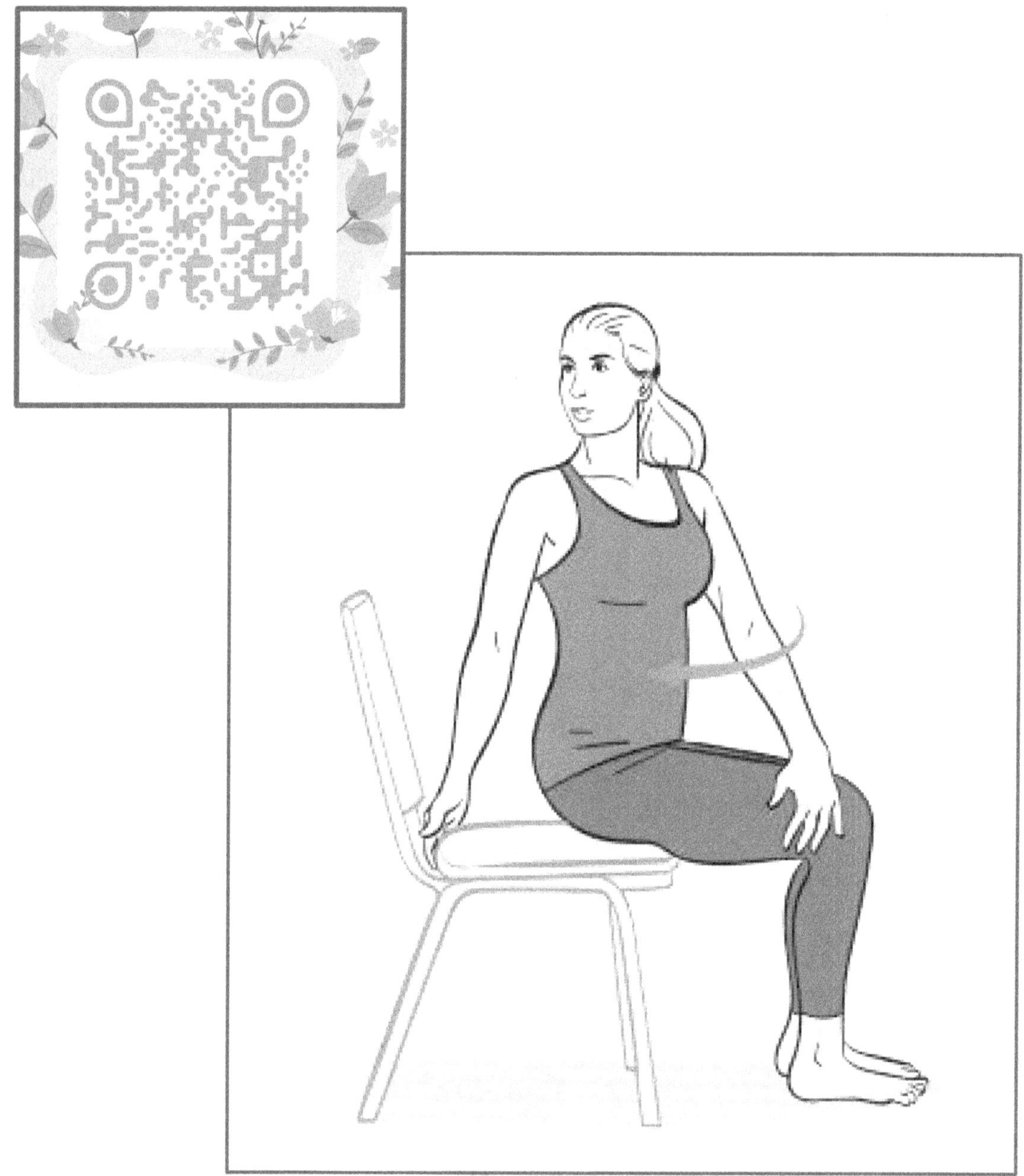

Seated Spinal Twist

Gentle Seated Backbend

The Gentle Seated Backbend is a calming pose that stretches the chest, shoulders, and abdomen. It's ideal for counteracting the effects of slouching and improving posture while energizing the body.

What You Need

- A sturdy chair with a backrest (optional).

Step-by-Step Instructions

Starting Position:

- Sit on the chair with your feet flat on the ground, hip-width apart.
- Place your hands on your thighs, keeping your spine long and shoulders relaxed.
- Begin the Backbend:
- Inhale deeply as you lift your chest upward and gently arch your upper back.
- Place your hands on the backrest of the chair for support, or keep them resting on your thighs if you prefer.

Lift the Gaze:

- Look upward or slightly ahead, keeping your neck long and avoiding compression.

- Hold the Pose:
- Hold the stretch for 3-5 breaths, feeling the gentle opening in your chest and shoulders.
- Release Slowly:
- Exhale as you return to an upright seated position.

Common Mistakes to Avoid

- Overarching the Lower Back: Focus the movement on your upper back and chest, not your lower back.
- Straining the Neck: Keep your neck aligned and avoid tilting it too far back.
- Collapsing the Core: Engage your abdominal muscles to support the backbend.

Benefits

- Opens the chest and improves breathing capacity.
- Relieves tension in the upper back and shoulders.
- Encourages better posture by counteracting slouching.
- Promotes relaxation and a feeling of lightness.

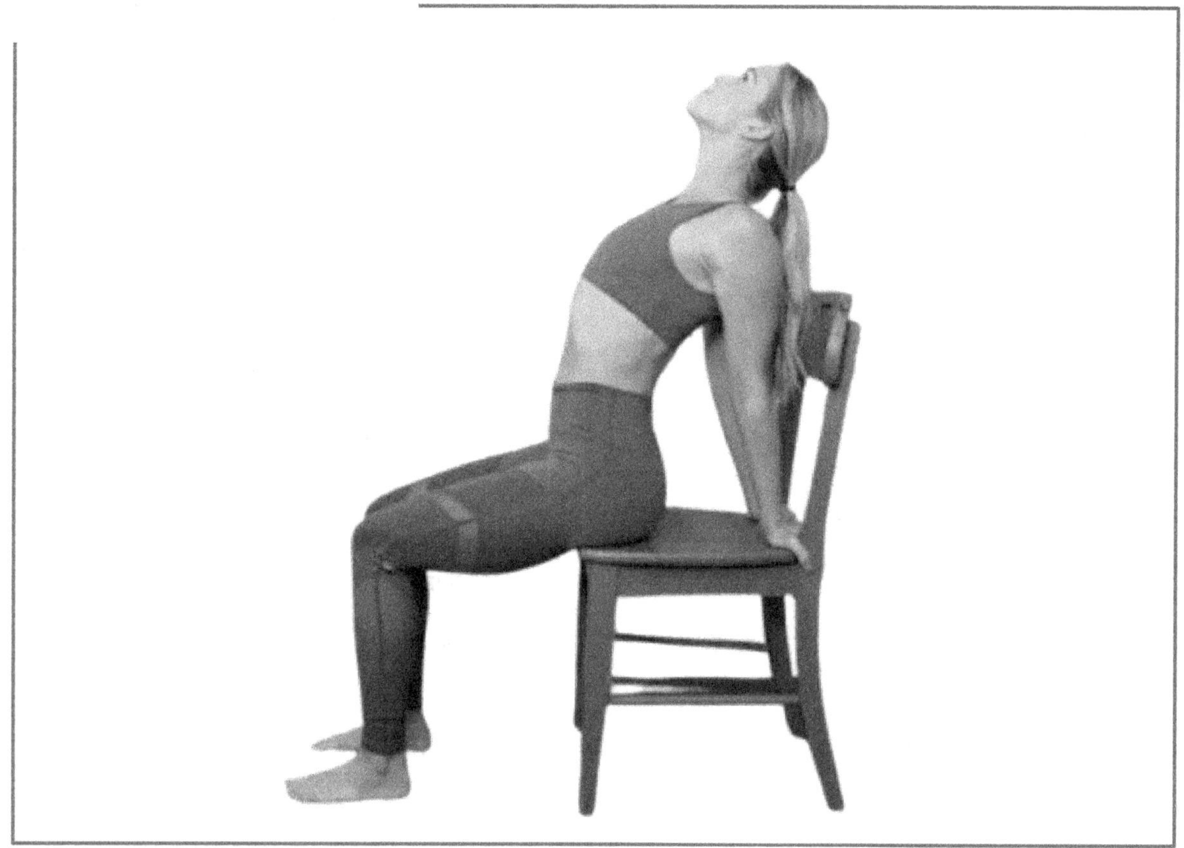

Gentle Seated Backbend

Midday Stretch for Tension Relief

Seated Pigeon Pose (for Hips)

The Seated Pigeon Pose is a hip-opening exercise that alleviates tightness in the hips and lower back. It's excellent for improving flexibility and mobility, especially for those who spend extended periods sitting.

What You Need

- A sturdy chair with no armrests.
- Optional: Cushion for added comfort under the hips.

Step-by-Step Instructions

Starting Position:

- Sit upright on the chair with your feet flat on the floor, hip-width apart.
- Position Your Leg:
- Lift your right leg and place your right ankle on your left thigh, just above the knee.
- Allow your right knee to drop naturally toward the floor, forming a "figure-four" shape with your legs.

Engage and Align:

- Flex your right foot to protect your knee joint.
- Sit tall and avoid slouching.
- Deepen the Stretch (Optional):
- If comfortable, hinge slightly forward at the hips while maintaining a straight back.
- Hold the position for 5-8 breaths, feeling the stretch in your right hip.

Switch Sides:

- Lower your right leg and repeat the pose on your left side.

Common Mistakes to Avoid

- Letting the Back Round: Keep your spine long and chest open.
- Forcing the Knee Down: Allow the knee to drop naturally without pressing it.
- Skipping Foot Flexion: Flexing the foot protects the knee and ensures proper alignment.

Benefits

- Releases tension in the hips and lower back.
- Improves hip flexibility and mobility.
- Alleviates discomfort caused by prolonged sitting.

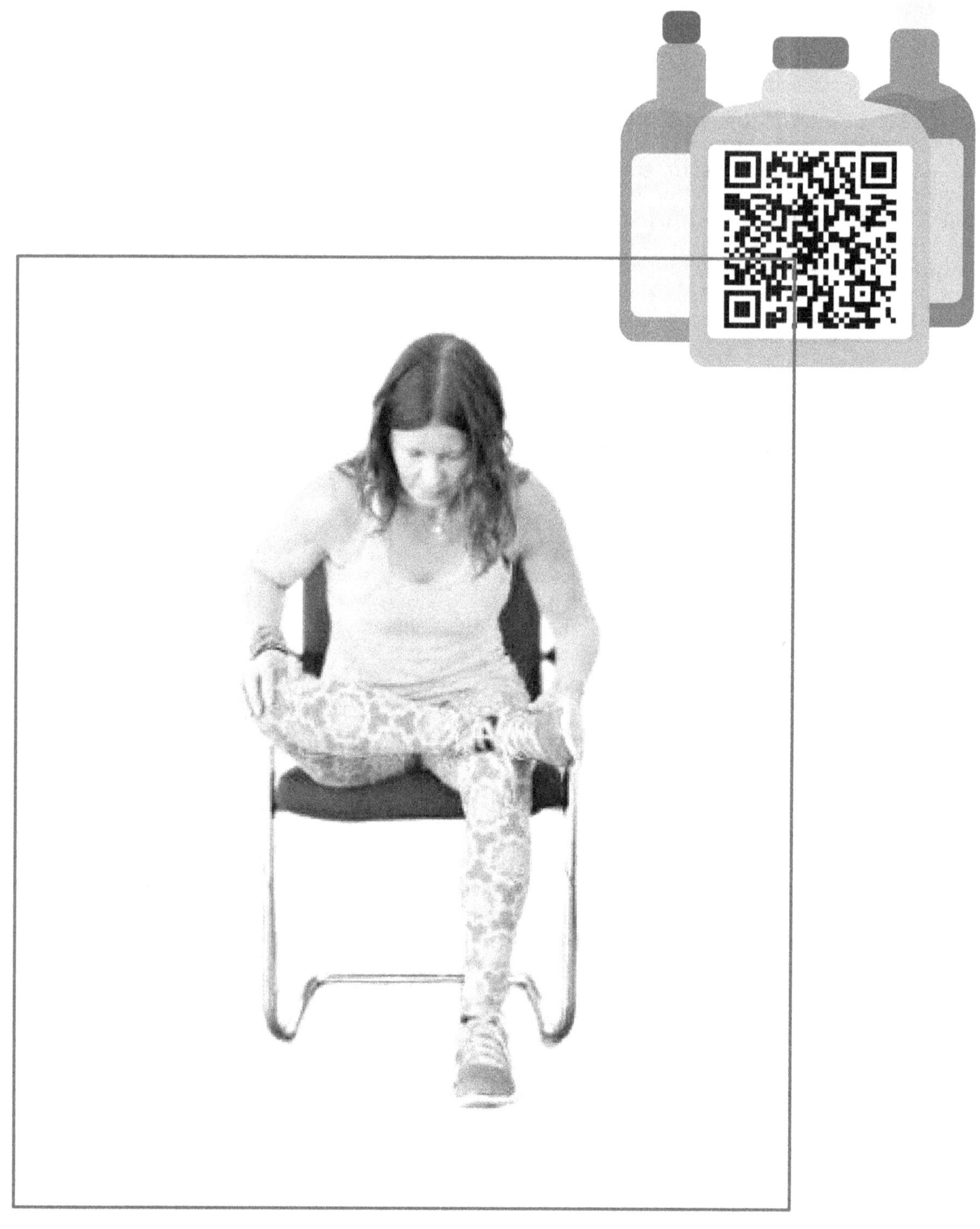

Seated Pigeon Pose (for Hips)

Chair Eagle Arms

Chair Eagle Arms stretches the shoulders, upper back, and arms while improving posture and flexibility. It's particularly helpful for releasing tension in the upper body.

What You Need

- A sturdy chair.

Step-by-Step Instructions

Starting Position:

- Sit tall with your feet flat on the floor.
- Extend both arms straight out in front of you at shoulder height.
- Cross Your Arms:
- Bring your right arm under your left arm, crossing at the elbows.

Bind the Arms (Optional):

- Bend both elbows, bringing the backs of your hands or palms together.
- If your palms don't touch, keep the backs of your hands together.
- Lift and Stretch:

- Inhale as you gently lift your elbows upward while keeping your shoulders relaxed.
- Hold the stretch for 5-8 breaths.

Switch Sides:

- Release the pose and repeat with your left arm under your right.

Common Mistakes to Avoid

- Tensing the Shoulders: Keep your shoulders relaxed, even as you lift your elbows.
- Forcing the Bind: If your hands don't meet, simply focus on the arm crossing.
- Rounding the Back: Sit tall to avoid slouching.

Benefits

- Stretches and strengthens the shoulders and upper back.
- Improves posture by counteracting slouching.
- Relieves tension caused by desk work or prolonged sitting.

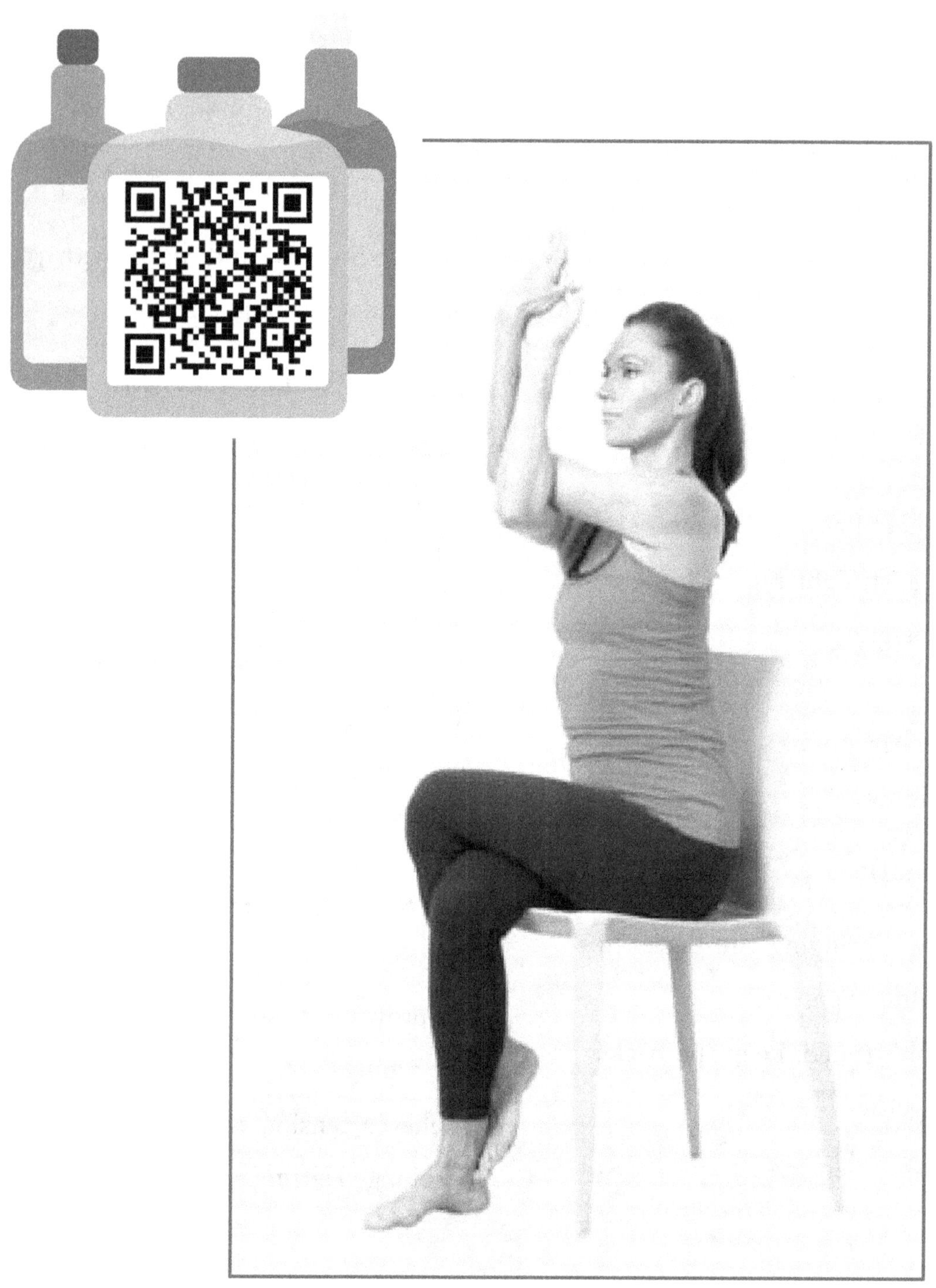

Chair Eagle Arms

Seated Hamstring Stretch

The Seated Hamstring Stretch gently elongates the hamstrings and lower back, enhancing flexibility and relieving tightness. This pose is great for improving range of motion and overall comfort.

What You Need

- A sturdy chair.
- Optional: Yoga strap or towel for extra support.

Step-by-Step Instructions

Starting Position:

- Sit on the edge of the chair with your feet flat on the floor.
- Extend Your Leg:
- Stretch your right leg straight out in front of you, placing your heel on the floor with your toes pointing upward.
- Keep your left foot flat on the floor.

Hinge at the Hips:

- Inhale as you lengthen your spine, then exhale as you hinge forward slightly from the hips.
- Rest your hands on your left thigh or gently reach toward your right toes.

Hold the Stretch:

- Feel the stretch along the back of your right leg.
- Hold for 5-8 breaths.

Switch Sides:

- Return to the starting position and repeat with your left leg.

Common Mistakes to Avoid

- Locking the Knee: Keep a slight bend in your extended leg to protect the joint.
- Rounding the Back: Focus on hinging from the hips rather than collapsing the spine.
- Overreaching: Stretch gently without forcing your hands to reach your toes.

Benefits

- Increases flexibility in the hamstrings and lower back.
- Alleviates tightness caused by prolonged sitting or standing.
- Improves range of motion and posture.

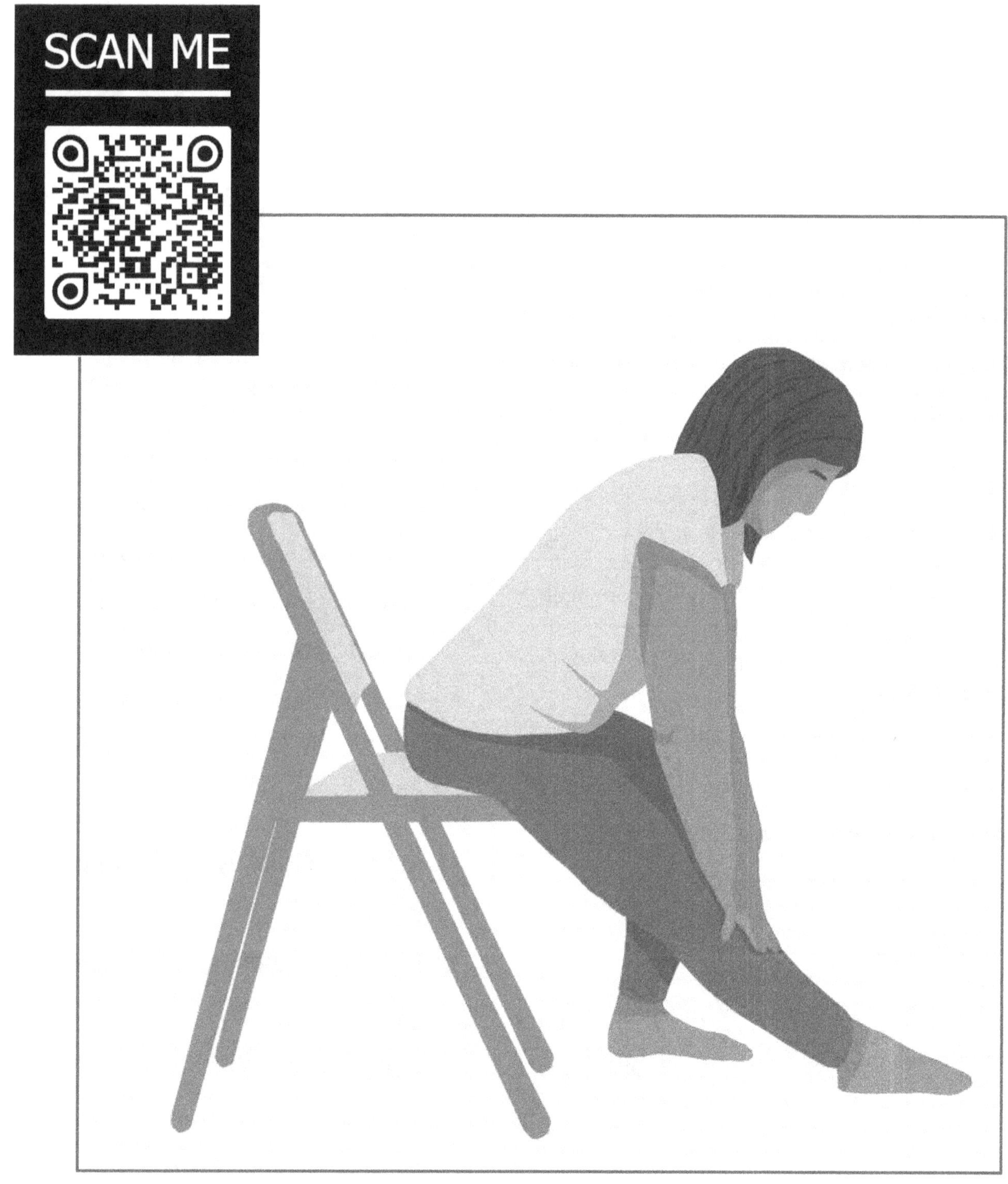

Seated Hamstring Stretch

Evening Flow for Relaxation

Seated Child's Pose

The Seated Child's Pose is a calming and restorative exercise that stretches the back, shoulders, and neck while promoting relaxation. It's perfect for winding down or relieving stress during the day.

What You Need

- A sturdy chair.
- Optional: Cushion for added comfort.

Step-by-Step Instructions

Starting Position:

- Sit comfortably on the chair with your feet flat on the floor, slightly apart.
- Rest your hands on your thighs.

Lean Forward:

- Slowly hinge forward at the hips, letting your chest come to rest on your thighs.
- Allow your hands to dangle toward the floor or rest them on your knees.

Rest Your Head:

Place your forehead on your hands, a cushion, or the back of another chair in front of you.

Relax and Breathe:

- Close your eyes and take deep, slow breaths.
- Hold this position for 5-8 breaths or as long as comfortable.

Return to Upright:

- Slowly roll up through your spine to return to a seated position.

Common Mistakes to Avoid

- Holding Your Breath: Focus on slow, steady breathing throughout.
- Tensing Shoulders: Keep your shoulders relaxed as you fold forward.
- Rushing Back Up: Take your time when returning to upright to avoid dizziness.

Benefits

- Relieves tension in the back and shoulders.
- Promotes relaxation and mental calmness.
- Gently stretches the spine and neck.

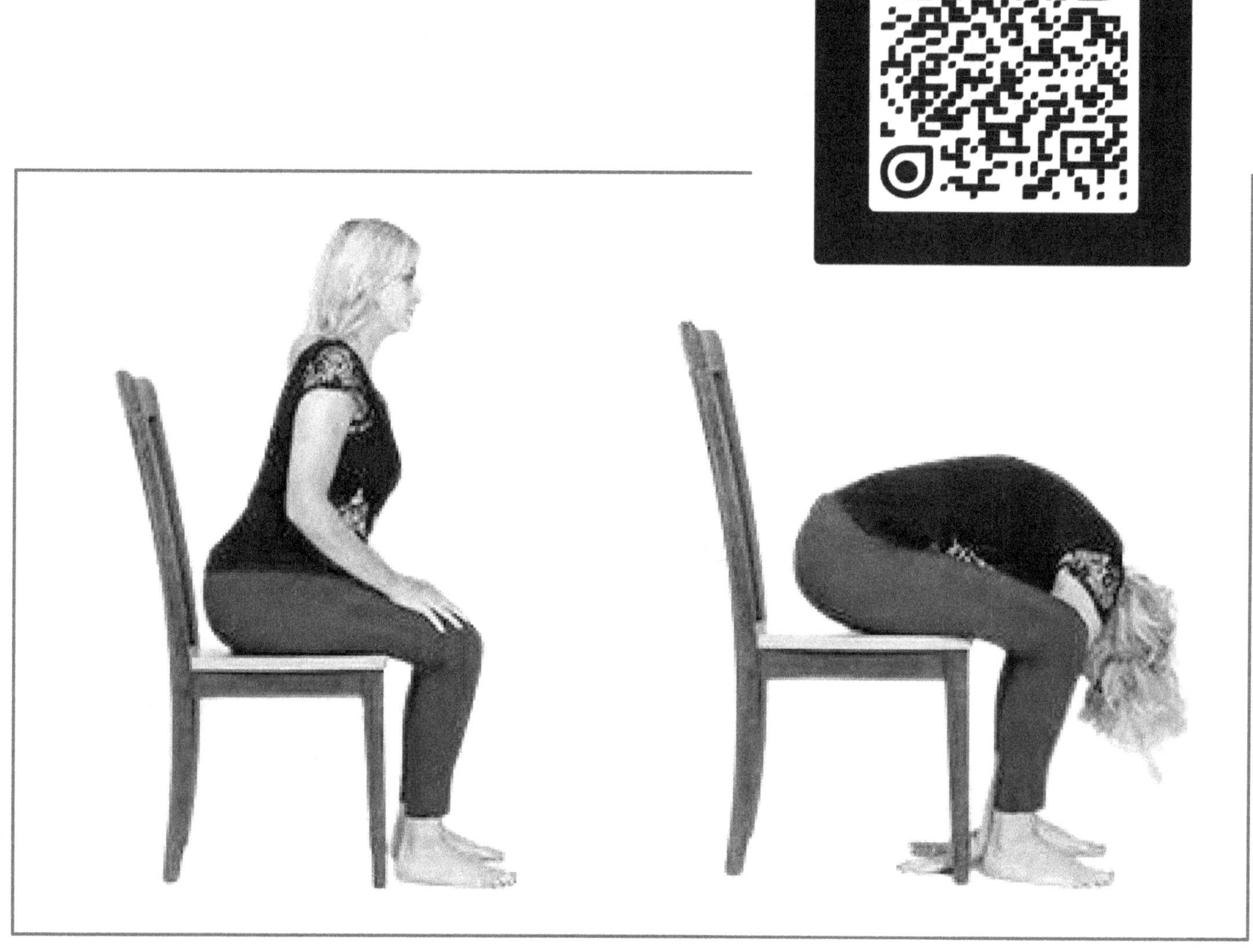

Seated Child's Pose

Gentle Seated Forward Fold with Breathing

This pose stretches the back, hamstrings, and shoulders while incorporating deep breathing for relaxation. It's an excellent way to decompress and release physical and mental stress.

What You Need

- A sturdy chair.

Step-by-Step Instructions

Starting Position:

- Sit on the edge of the chair with your feet flat on the floor and knees hip-width apart.

Fold Forward:

- Inhale to lengthen your spine, then exhale as you hinge forward at the hips.
- Let your arms dangle toward the floor, or rest them on your thighs.

Deep Breathing:

- Inhale deeply through your nose and exhale slowly through your mouth.
- Hold the pose for 5-10 breaths, feeling the stretch along your back and legs.

Return to Upright:

- Slowly roll up through your spine, stacking each vertebra until you are sitting tall again.

Common Mistakes to Avoid

- Rounding the Back Too Much: Focus on hinging at the hips rather than collapsing the spine.
- Shallow Breathing: Take slow, deep breaths to enhance relaxation.
- Overstretching: Go as far as comfortable without straining.

Benefits

Stretches the spine, hamstrings, and shoulders.

Encourages mindful breathing and relaxation.

Relieves tension and improves flexibility.

SCAN QR CODE FOR EXERCISE VIDEOS

SCAN ME

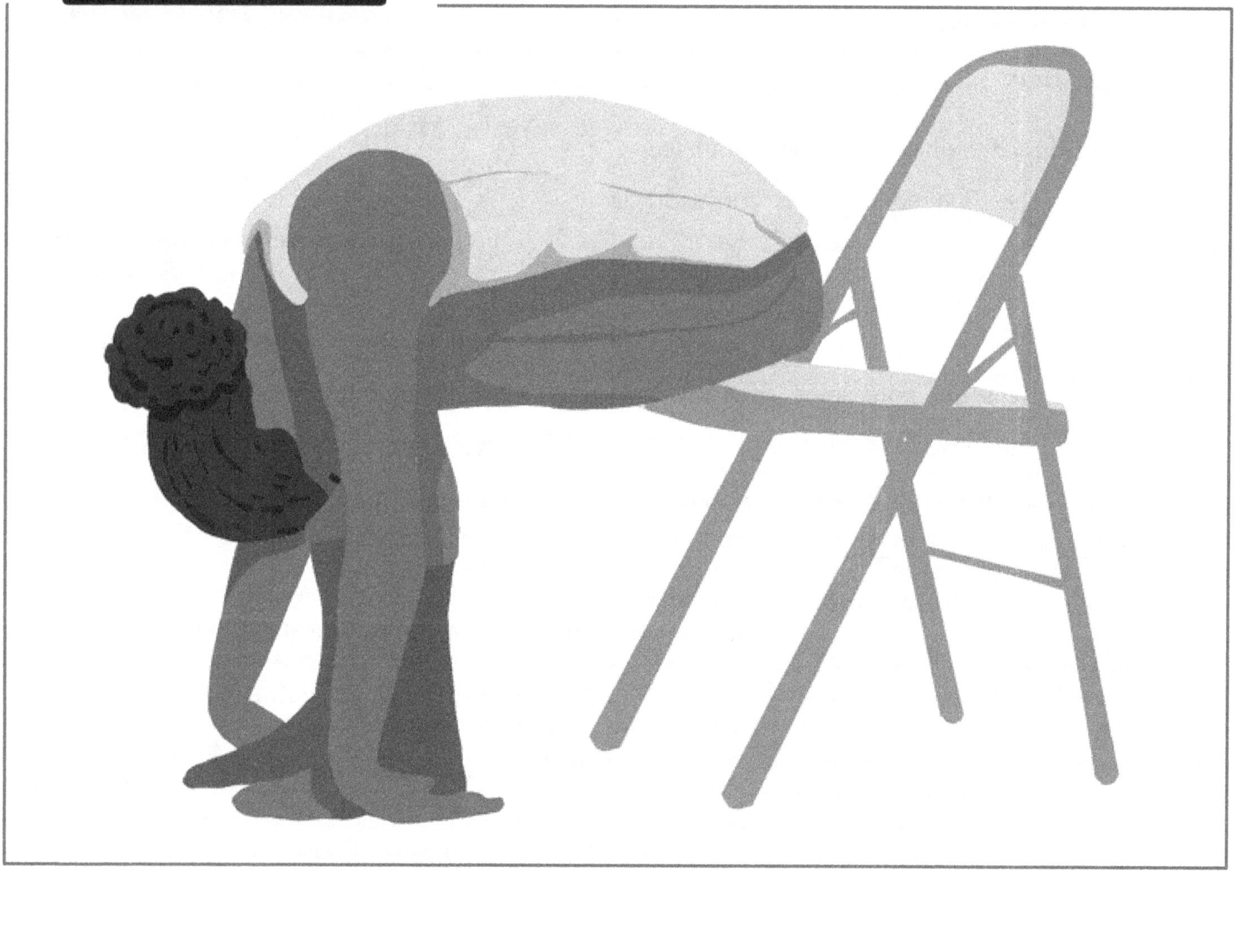

Guided Relaxation with Seated Breathing

Guided Relaxation with Seated Breathing combines mindfulness and gentle breathing techniques to reduce stress, improve focus, and create a sense of calm. It's a perfect way to end your chair yoga practice.

What You Need

- A sturdy chair.
- Optional: Soft music or a timer for guidance.

Step-by-Step Instructions

Starting Position:

- Sit comfortably on the chair with your feet flat on the floor.
- Rest your hands on your thighs or place them gently in your lap.

Close Your Eyes:

- Allow your eyes to close or soften your gaze.

Focus on Your Breathing:

- Inhale deeply through your nose for a count of four.
- Hold your breath for a count of two.
- Exhale slowly through your mouth for a count of six.

Visualize Relaxation:

- Imagine a wave of relaxation starting at your head and flowing down to your toes with each exhale.

Continue for a Few Minutes:

- Repeat the breathing cycle for 2-5 minutes, or as desired.
- Gently Return to Awareness:
- Open your eyes and stretch your arms lightly overhead to complete the practice.

Common Mistakes to Avoid

- Shallow Breathing: Ensure each inhale and exhale is deep and controlled.
- Tension in the Body: Relax your shoulders and jaw as you breathe.
- Rushing the Process: Allow yourself to take your time and enjoy the calm.

Benefits

Reduces stress and anxiety.

Improves focus and mindfulness.

Promotes a sense of overall well-being and relaxation.

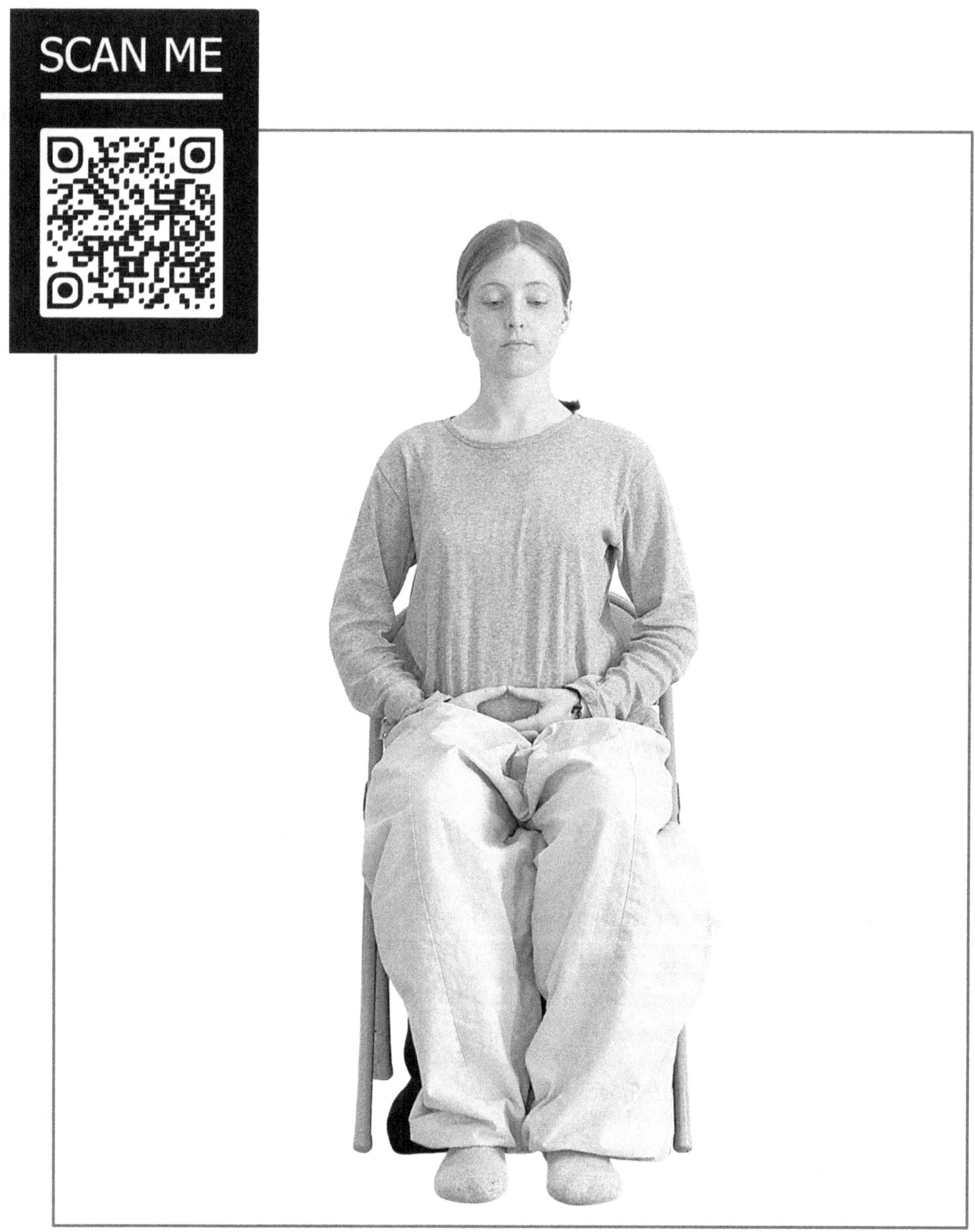

Guided Relaxation with Seated Breathing

Fun Challenges to Try Daily

Chair Yoga Daily Fun Challenges Tracker

Track your progress and stay motivated with this printable guide to daily chair yoga challenges. Each challenge is designed to help you improve flexibility, strength, and mindfulness while keeping your routine fun and engaging.

Challenge 1: The Flexibility Test

Exercise: Gentle Seated Forward Fold with Breathing

- **Goal:** Stretch a little deeper each day.

- **Tracking:** Mark how close your hands come to your toes each day.

Day	Can I reach closer to my toes? (Y/N)	Notes
Day 1		
Day 2		
Day 3		
Day 4		
Day 5		

Challenge 2: Balance and Core Stability

Exercise: Seated Pigeon Pose

- **Goal:** Hold the pose for 10 seconds longer each day.

- **Tracking:** Record how steady you feel.

Day	Seconds Held	How Steady Did I Feel? (1-10)	Notes
Day 1			
Day 2			
Day 3			
Day 4			
Day 5			

Challenge 3: Endurance Flow

Exercise: Seated Sun Salutation

- **Goal:** Add one extra repetition each day.

- **Tracking:** Note how many rounds you completed.

Day	Rounds Completed	How Did I Feel? (1-10)	Notes
Day 1			
Day 2			
Day 3			
Day 4			
Day 5			

Challenge 4: Breath Control Mastery

Exercise: Gentle Seated Forward Fold with Breathing

- **Goal:** Extend your exhale by one second each day.

- **Tracking:** Record the number of seconds for each exhale.

Day	Seconds for Exhale	How Relaxed Did I Feel? (1-10)	Notes
Day 1			
Day 2			
Day 3			
Day 4			
Day 5			

Challenge 5: Pose Customization 🎨✨🪑

Exercise: Create a mini-flow using Seated Shoulder Rolls, Wrist and Ankle Rotations, and Chair Warrior II.

- **Goal:** Personalize your yoga routine by experimenting with flow combinations.

- **Tracking:** Write down your flow combination and rate how it felt.

Day	Flow Combination	How Did It Feel? (1-10)	Notes
Day 1			
Day 2			
Day 3			
Day 4			
Day 5			

Challenge 6: Morning Motivation 🪦☀️❓

Exercise: Start your day with Seated Sun Salutation and Gentle Seated Backbend.

- **Goal:** Rate your energy before and after the routine.

- **Tracking:** Use the table to track your energy levels.

Day	Energy Before (1-10)	Energy After (1-10)	Notes
Day 1			
Day 2			
Day 3			
Day 4			
Day 5			

Challenge 7: Nighttime Wind-Down 🌙🛏️🌸

Exercise: Seated Child's Pose and Guided Relaxation with Breathing

- **Goal:** Extend the duration of each pose nightly.

- **Tracking:** Record how long you held the pose and how relaxed you felt.

Day	Pose	Duration (Minutes)	Relaxation Level (1-10)	Notes
Day 1				
Day 2				
Day 3				
Day 4				
Day 5				

Part 3: Chair Yoga for Weight Loss

Seated Marching with Arm Lifts

This dynamic exercise increases your heart rate, burns calories, and strengthens both upper and lower body muscles.

Equipment Needed:

- A sturdy chair with no wheels and enough room for arm movements.

Step-by-Step Instructions:

- Sit upright with your feet flat on the ground, hip-width apart.
- Start marching by lifting one knee at a time toward your chest, alternating legs.
- Simultaneously, raise both arms overhead as if reaching for the ceiling.
- Lower your arms as you lower each leg and repeat the movement.
- Continue for 1 minute or more, gradually increasing your speed as you feel comfortable.

Common Mistakes to Avoid:

- Slouching while marching—engage your core to maintain an upright posture.
- Overextending your arm lifts, can strain your shoulders.

Benefits:

- Boosts heart rate for calorie burn.
- Strengthens core, leg, and arm muscles.
- Improves coordination and endurance.

SCAN QR CODE FOR EXERCISE VIDEOS

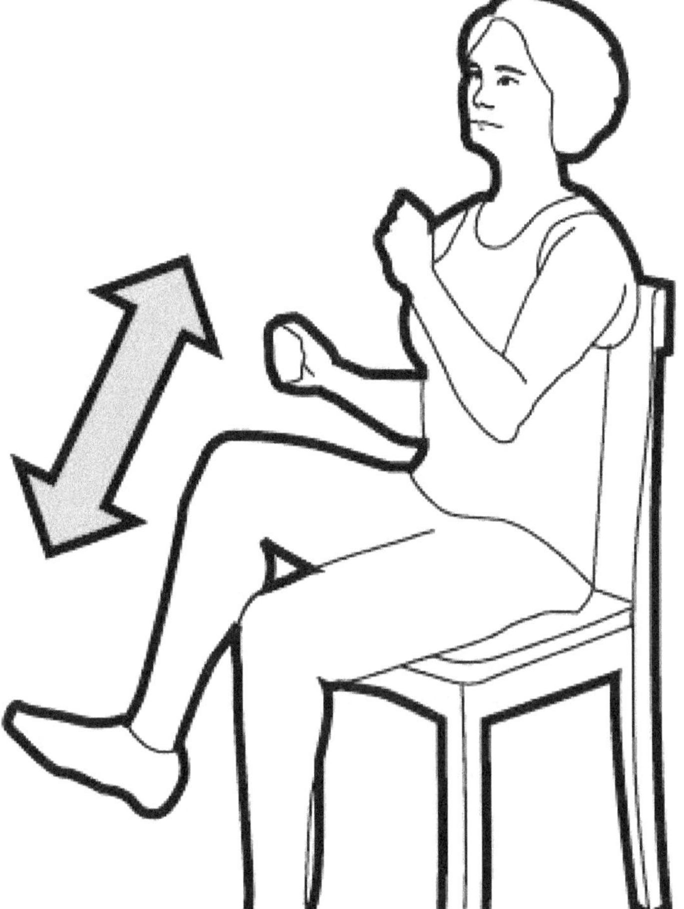

Chair Push-Ups (Using the Chair for Support)

Chair push-ups are a low-impact way to tone your arms, shoulders, and chest while also engaging your core.

Equipment Needed:

- A stable chair that won't slide on the floor.

Step-by-Step Instructions:

- Sit on the edge of the chair with your feet firmly planted on the floor.
- Place your hands on the edge of the seat, fingers pointing forward, and shift your weight onto your arms.
- Walk your feet slightly forward, keeping your knees bent.
- Lower your body by bending your elbows, keeping them close to your sides.
- Push yourself back up to the starting position.
- Repeat for 8–12 reps.

Common Mistakes to Avoid:

- Letting your shoulders shrug—keep them down and away from your ears.
- Using momentum instead of controlled movements.

Benefits:

- Strengthens arm, chest, and shoulder muscles.
- Engages the core for stability.
- Increases upper body endurance.

SCAN QR CODE FOR EXERCISE VIDEOS

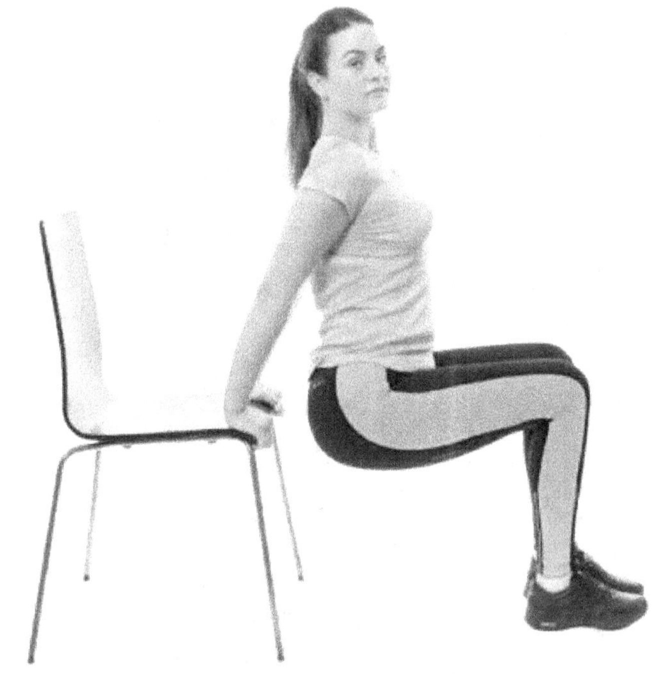

Core Strengthening Forward Fold

This move is excellent for engaging your abdominal muscles while stretching your back and hamstrings. It combines core strengthening with flexibility, making it a balanced addition to your routine.

Equipment Needed:

- A sturdy chair without wheels.

Step-by-Step Instructions:

- Sit tall on the chair with your feet flat on the floor, hip-width apart.
- Place your hands on your thighs or extend them forward for a deeper stretch.
- Engage your core by gently pulling your navel toward your spine.
- Slowly hinge forward at the hips, keeping your back straight, until your torso comes close to your thighs.
- Hold for 3-5 seconds, then use your core muscles to return to an upright position.
- Repeat 8-10 times.

Common Mistakes to Avoid:

- Rounding your back while folding forward.
- Letting your shoulders hunch up toward your ears.
- Forgetting to engage your core muscles.

Benefits:

- Strengthens the core muscles.
- Improves spinal flexibility.
- Gently stretches the back and hamstrings.

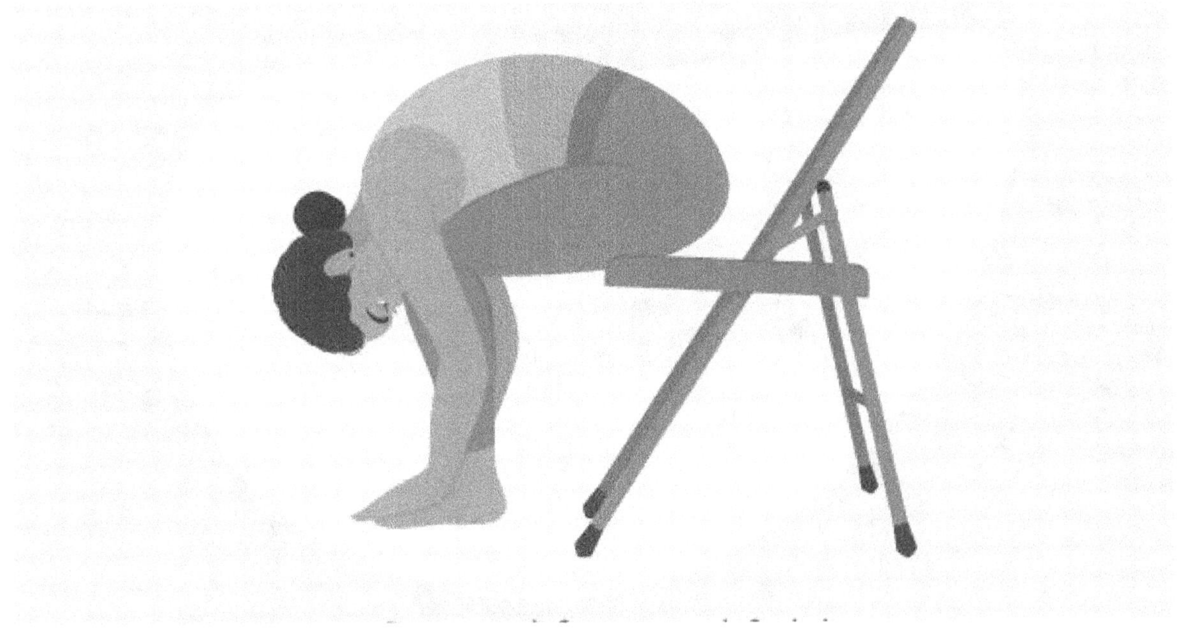

Seated Knee-to-Elbow Crunches

This dynamic exercise targets the obliques and lower abs while improving coordination and mobility. It's a fun and engaging way to work on your core strength.

Equipment Needed:

- A sturdy chair without armrests.

Step-by-Step Instructions:

- Sit on the edge of the chair with your back straight and feet flat on the floor.
- Place your hands lightly behind your head, elbows wide.
- Lift your right knee toward your chest while simultaneously twisting your torso to bring your left elbow toward the knee.
- Return to the starting position and repeat on the other side, bringing your right elbow to your left knee.
- Continue alternating sides for 10-12 repetitions per side.

Common Mistakes to Avoid:

- Pulling on your neck instead of using your core muscles.

- Letting your back slump or shoulders round forward.

- Rushing through the movements without proper form.

Benefits:

- Tones the obliques and lower abs.

- Improves coordination and balance.

- Encourages spinal mobility.

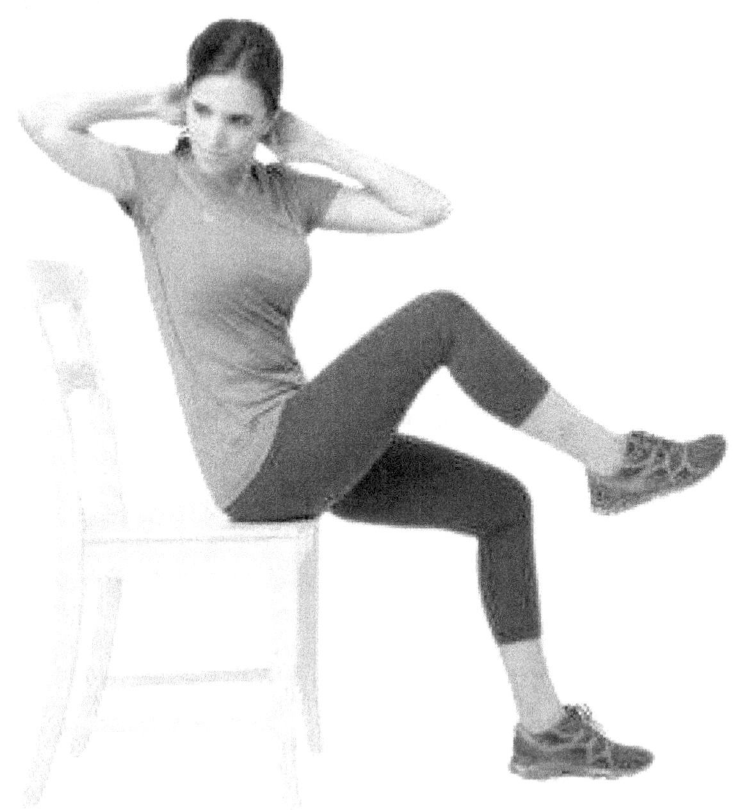

Seated Side Plank Pose (Modified)

This modified version of a side plank strengthens your obliques, shoulders, and core while being accessible for chair yoga practitioners.

Equipment Needed:

- A sturdy chair with no wheels.

Step-by-Step Instructions:

1. Sit sideways on the chair with your left side close to the chair back and feet flat on the floor.

2. Place your left hand on the chair seat for support.

3. Extend your right leg out to the side, keeping it straight and your right foot on the floor.

4. Lift your right arm overhead, creating a long line from your fingertips to your extended foot.

5. Engage your core and hold this position for 5-10 seconds.

6. Slowly return to the starting position and repeat on the other side.

Common Mistakes to Avoid:

- Letting your hips sag or rotate forward.

- Overextending your supporting arm, which can strain your shoulder.

- Forgetting to keep your core engaged.

Benefits:

- Strengthens the obliques and core.

- Builds shoulder stability.

- Enhances balance and posture.

SCAN QR CODE FOR EXERCISE VIDEOS

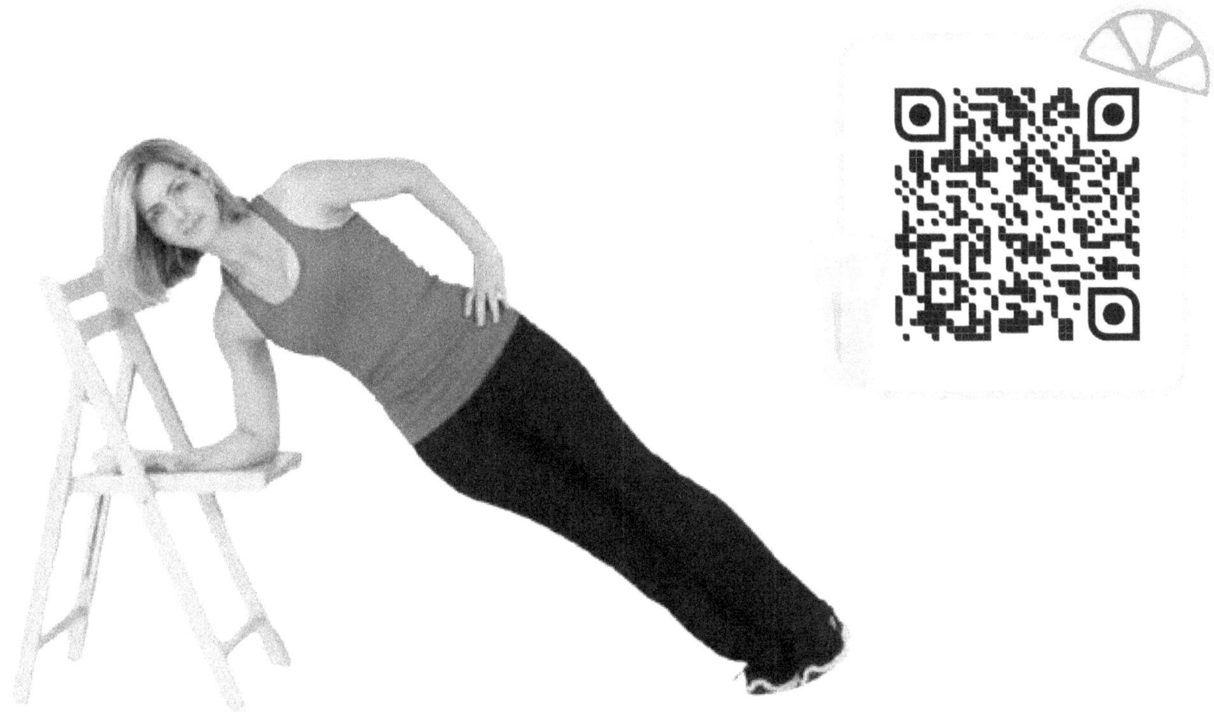

Chair Arm Circles (Weighted Optional)

This exercise helps tone your shoulders and improve arm mobility. Using light weights adds an extra challenge for strength building.

Equipment Needed:

- A sturdy chair without wheels.

- Optional: Light weights (1–3 pounds) or small water bottles.

Step-by-Step Instructions:

1. Sit upright in the chair with feet flat on the floor and back straight.

2. Extend both arms out to the sides at shoulder height, palms facing downward.

3. Begin making small circles with your arms, moving them forward for 10-12 seconds.

4. Reverse the motion, circling your arms backward for another 10-12 seconds.

5. If using weights, hold them securely in your hands while performing the motion.

6. Repeat for 2-3 sets, resting between rounds if needed.

Common Mistakes to Avoid:

- Letting your shoulders rise toward your ears.

- Losing control of the circular motion.

- Holding your breath; maintain steady breathing.

Benefits:

- Strengthens shoulders and upper arms.

- Improves arm flexibility and mobility.

- Can enhance posture over time.

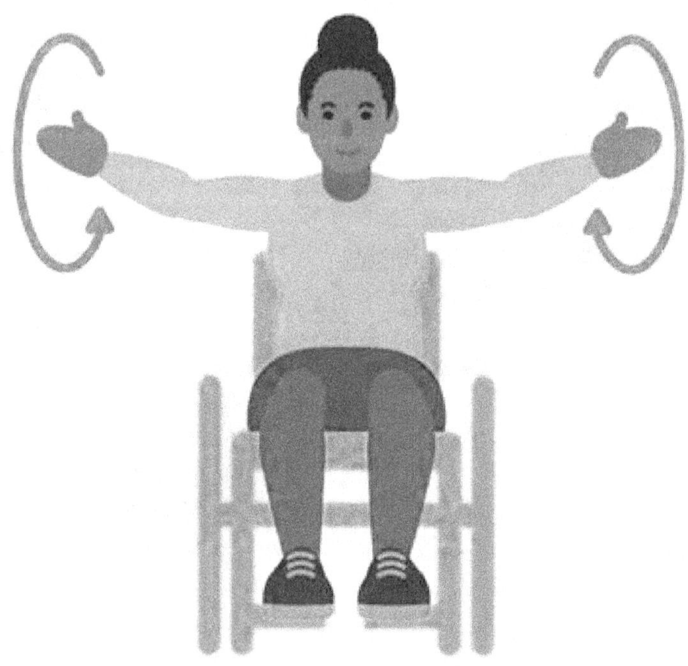

Seated Heel Raises for Calf Toning

This simple but effective exercise strengthens and tones your calves while improving circulation in the legs.

Equipment Needed:

- A sturdy chair without wheels.

Step-by-Step Instructions:

1. Sit tall with your feet flat on the floor and hands resting on your thighs or chair armrests for support.

2. Slowly lift both heels off the floor, balancing on the balls of your feet.

3. Hold the raised position for 2-3 seconds.

4. Lower your heels back down slowly and with control.

5. Repeat for 12-15 repetitions, aiming for 2-3 sets.

Common Mistakes to Avoid:

- Letting your knees wobble inward or outward.

- Bouncing up and down instead of moving with control.

- Forgetting to keep your core engaged and back straight.

Benefits:

- Strengthens calf muscles.

- Enhances lower leg endurance and stability.

- Improves blood circulation in the feet and ankles.

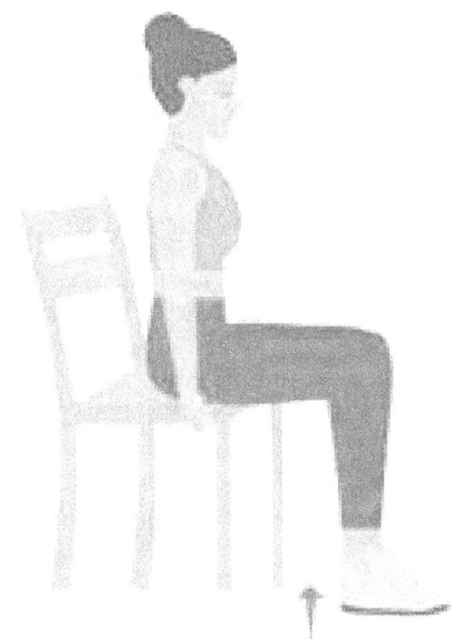

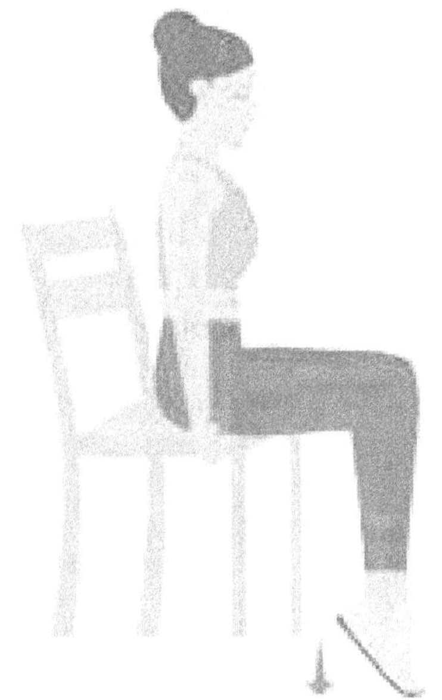

Chair Yoga for Arthritis Relief

Chair yoga can offer relief to arthritis sufferers by promoting joint flexibility, reducing stiffness, and improving circulation. These gentle movements are tailored to be safe and effective for those with joint pain or limited mobility.

Gentle Wrist Rolls and Hand Stretches

This exercise focuses on easing tension and improving mobility in the wrists and hands, areas often affected by arthritis.

Equipment Needed:

- A sturdy chair without wheels.

Step-by-Step Instructions:

1. Sit comfortably with your back straight and feet flat on the floor.

2. Extend your arms forward, palms facing down.

3. Slowly rotate your wrists in a circular motion, clockwise for 10 seconds.

4. Reverse the direction, moving counterclockwise for another 10 seconds.

5. Interlace your fingers, then gently stretch your hands forward, palms facing outward. Hold for 5 seconds.

6. Release and shake out your hands to relax them.

7. Repeat the sequence 2-3 times.

Common Mistakes to Avoid:

- Moving too quickly; prioritize slow, controlled movements.

- Skipping the stretch after the rolls.

- Overextending the wrists, which can cause discomfort.

Benefits:

- Enhances wrist and finger flexibility.

- Relieves stiffness in hands and forearms.

- Improves circulation to joints and tendons.

Seated Neck and Shoulder Stretches

This stretch alleviates tension in the neck and shoulders, common areas for arthritis discomfort, while enhancing flexibility and promoting relaxation.

Equipment Needed:

- A sturdy chair without wheels.

Step-by-Step Instructions:

1. Sit tall with your feet flat on the floor, hands resting on your thighs.

2. Gently tilt your head to the right, bringing your right ear toward your right shoulder. Hold for 5-10 seconds.

3. Return to center and repeat on the left side.

4. Lower your chin toward your chest, feeling a stretch along the back of your neck. Hold for 5-10 seconds.

5. Raise your head and gently roll your shoulders backward in a circular motion for 10 seconds.

6. Repeat the shoulder rolls forward for 10 seconds.

7. Perform the sequence 2-3 times.

Common Mistakes to Avoid:

- Forcing your head or shoulders beyond their comfortable range of motion.

- Slouching while performing the stretches.

- Holding your breath; maintain steady breathing.

Benefits:

- Relieves tension and stiffness in the neck and shoulders.

- Improves joint mobility and posture.

- Promotes relaxation and reduces stress.

Stress-Relief Flow to Reduce Emotional Eating

This sequence is designed to alleviate stress and create a sense of calm, which can help break the cycle of emotional eating. By combining gentle movement, focused breathing, and mindfulness, this flow soothes the body and mind, reducing the urge to turn to food for comfort.

Chair Cat-Cow Stretch

A gentle movement to release tension in the spine and stimulate circulation, helping to calm the nervous system.

Equipment Needed:

- A sturdy chair without wheels.

Step-by-Step Instructions:

1. Sit on the edge of the chair with your feet flat on the floor, hands resting on your knees.

2. **Cow Pose:** Inhale as you arch your back, rolling your shoulders back and lifting your chest toward the ceiling. Let your head follow the movement, tilting slightly upward.

3. **Cat Pose:** Exhale as you round your spine, tucking your chin toward your chest and pulling your belly button in.

4. Flow between Cat and Cow poses with each inhale and exhale for 8-10 cycles.

Common Mistakes to Avoid:

- Holding your breath; ensure each movement is tied to your breathing.

- Slumping or forcing the movement beyond your comfort zone.

Benefits:

- Relieves stress and tension in the back and shoulders.

- Promotes mindful breathing and relaxation.

- Enhances spinal flexibility.

Seated Breathing and Visualization

This practice helps calm the mind and shift focus away from stressors by incorporating guided imagery with breathing techniques.

Equipment Needed:

- A sturdy chair without wheels.

Step-by-Step Instructions:

1. Sit upright with your hands resting on your thighs or in your lap.

2. Close your eyes and take a deep inhale through your nose, expanding your belly.

3. Exhale slowly through your mouth, releasing tension.

4. Visualize a calming scene, such as a peaceful beach or a quiet forest.

5. Continue to breathe deeply, imagining yourself in this serene space for 2-3 minutes.

6. Open your eyes slowly and take one final deep breath before resuming your day.

Common Mistakes to Avoid:

- Shallow breathing; aim for slow, deep breaths.

- Letting your mind wander; gently bring focus back to your visualization if needed.

Benefits:

- Reduces stress and calms the mind.

- Improves focus and emotional control.

- Encourages mindful awareness of cravings and triggers.

Guided Seated Meditation

A mindfulness practice to promote relaxation and awareness, helping you reconnect with your body's hunger and fullness cues.

Equipment Needed:

- A sturdy chair without wheels.

- Optional: Soothing music or a meditation app.

Step-by-Step Instructions:

1. Sit with your back straight, feet flat on the floor, and hands resting on your lap.

2. Close your eyes and take a few deep breaths, allowing your body to relax.

3. Bring your attention to your breath, noticing the inhale and exhale without changing it.

4. If your mind wanders, gently bring your focus back to your breath.

5. After 3-5 minutes, take a final deep breath and slowly open your eyes.

Common Mistakes to Avoid:

- Becoming frustrated if your mind wanders; this is natural and part of the process.

- Forcing yourself to sit longer than feels comfortable; consistency matters more than duration.

Benefits:

- Promotes relaxation and reduces emotional triggers.

- Builds awareness of emotional eating patterns.

- Encourages mindfulness and self-compassion.

These workouts are designed to elevate your heart rate and boost your energy without needing to leave your chair. Perfect for improving cardiovascular health, burning calories, and keeping your routine fun and engaging.

Seated Boxing Punches

This exercise mimics the movements of boxing to provide a low-impact cardio boost while strengthening your arms and shoulders.

Equipment Needed:

- A sturdy chair without wheels.

- Optional: Light hand weights or resistance bands for added intensity.

Step-by-Step Instructions:

1. Sit up straight on your chair with your feet flat on the floor, shoulder-width apart.

2. Make loose fists with both hands and bring them up to chest height, elbows bent.

3. Extend your right arm straight forward as if throwing a punch, keeping your fist at shoulder height.

4. Retract your right arm and immediately punch forward with your left arm.

5. Alternate punches at a steady pace for 1-2 minutes, increasing speed as you feel comfortable.

Common Mistakes to Avoid:

- Overextending your elbows; keep a slight bend in your arms.

- Slouching or leaning back; maintain an upright posture.

Benefits:

- Boosts heart rate for a quick cardio session.

- Strengthens the arms, shoulders, and core.

- Improves coordination and endurance.

Seated Marching with Arm Movements

This exercise combines leg and arm movements to provide a full-body cardio workout while seated.

Equipment Needed:

- A sturdy chair without wheels.

Step-by-Step Instructions:

1. Sit with your back straight and feet flat on the floor.

2. Lift your right knee as high as possible while simultaneously raising your left arm overhead.

3. Lower your leg and arm and immediately repeat with your left knee and right arm.

4. Continue alternating sides in a marching motion for 1-2 minutes, gradually increasing your speed.

Common Mistakes to Avoid:

- Forgetting to engage your core; keep it active for stability.

- Letting your shoulders tense up; keep them relaxed.

Benefits:

- Increases heart rate for calorie-burning cardio.

- Strengthens leg and arm muscles.

- Improves coordination and rhythm.

Chair Jumping Jacks (Arms Only)

A seated version of the classic jumping jack that focuses on arm movements to get your blood flowing.

Equipment Needed:

- A sturdy chair without wheels.

Step-by-Step Instructions:

1. Sit upright on the chair with your feet flat on the floor and arms resting at your sides.

2. Raise both arms out to the sides and up overhead, clapping your hands together if possible.

3. Lower your arms back to the starting position and repeat.

4. Perform the movement quickly for 1-2 minutes to keep your heart rate elevated.

Common Mistakes to Avoid:

- Using momentum rather than controlled arm movements.

- Slouching or leaning forward; maintain a tall, upright posture.

Benefits:

- Provides a low-impact cardio workout.

- Strengthens the shoulders and improves mobility.

- Easy to adapt for various fitness levels.

Mindfulness and Breathing Techniques

To fully benefit from chair yoga, integrating mindfulness and breathing techniques can enhance relaxation, focus, and overall well-being. This section introduces deep breathing exercises and visualization practices to reduce stress and deepen your connection to your practice.

Deep Breathing Exercises

Deep breathing activates the parasympathetic nervous system, promoting relaxation and reducing stress. It's a simple yet powerful way to center your mind and body.

Equipment Needed:

- A sturdy chair with a backrest for support.

Step-by-Step Instructions:

1. Sit comfortably with your back straight and feet flat on the floor. Rest your hands on your thighs.
2. Inhale deeply through your nose, allowing your belly to expand as you fill your lungs with air. Count to 4 as you inhale.
3. Hold your breath for a count of 4, keeping your body relaxed.
4. Slowly exhale through your mouth for a count of 6, allowing your belly to deflate completely.
5. Repeat this cycle for 5-10 minutes, gradually increasing the duration as you become more comfortable.

Common Mistakes to Avoid:

- Breathing shallowly into your chest rather than deeply into your belly.
- Tensing your shoulders or jaw; keep them relaxed.

Benefits:

- Reduces stress and anxiety.
- Improves lung capacity and oxygen flow.
- Enhances focus and mindfulness.

Visualization for Stress Reduction

Visualization combines mental imagery with deep breathing to calm the mind and create a sense of peace. It's a helpful tool for managing stress and cultivating positivity.

Equipment Needed:

- A quiet space with a comfortable chair.

Step-by-Step Instructions:

1. Sit comfortably with your feet flat on the floor and hands resting on your thighs.

2. Close your eyes and take a few deep breaths, inhaling through your nose and exhaling through your mouth.

3. Imagine a peaceful scene, such as a serene beach, a lush forest, or a cozy room.

4. Engage your senses: picture the colors, hear the sounds, feel the textures, and even smell the scents of your imagined setting.

5. As you visualize, synchronize your breathing to the rhythm of your scene. For example, imagine waves gently rolling in as you inhale and receding as you exhale.

6. Continue for 5-10 minutes, gradually returning your awareness to the present moment.

Common Mistakes to Avoid:

- Forcing an image to appear; let your imagination flow naturally.
- Allowing distractions to break your focus; gently bring your mind back to the scene if it wanders.

Benefits:

- Eases tension and stress.
- Promotes mental clarity and relaxation.
- Encourages a positive mindset.

FAQs and Troubleshooting Common Challenges

What if I can't complete the 15 minutes?

It's okay! Consistency matters more than duration. Start with just 5 or 10 minutes a day and gradually increase your time. Remember, even small efforts make a big difference. Focus on quality over quantity, and celebrate your progress. 🎉

How do I manage discomfort during poses?

Discomfort is different from pain. If a pose feels too challenging, try a modification or adjust your position. Use props like cushions or a rolled towel for extra support. Listen to your body—if something feels wrong, pause and reset. 💡

Can I do this with [specific condition]?

Chair yoga is generally gentle and adaptable for many conditions, but it's always best to consult your healthcare provider before starting. Tailor poses to your comfort level and avoid movements that exacerbate your symptoms.

Adjusting Intensity Levels

For Beginners:

- Focus on slow, controlled movements.
- Take breaks as needed and prioritize gentle poses like Seated Breathing and Gentle Wrist Rolls.
- Use props to enhance support and stability.

For Advanced Users:

- Add light weights or resistance bands to increase challenge.
- Hold poses for longer durations or increase repetitions.
- Combine multiple poses into a seamless flow for a more dynamic practice.

Modifications for Beginners and Advanced Users

Beginner Modifications:

- **Seated Forward Fold:** Keep hands on your thighs instead of reaching for your toes.
- **Chair Warrior II:** Rest your hands on the chair for added balance.
- **Seated Pigeon Pose:** Cross one leg loosely and avoid pressing too deeply.

Advanced Modifications:

- **Chair Push-Ups:** Perform a greater range of motion or add a light weight on your lap.
- **Seated Side Plank Pose:** Extend your arm upward and hold the pose longer.
- **Chair Jumping Jacks:** Use light weights for added resistance.

How to Incorporate Chair Yoga into Daily Life

TV Time:

During commercial breaks or favorite shows, do quick exercises like Seated Shoulder Rolls or Wrist and Ankle Rotations.

Work Breaks:

Take 5-10 minutes to stretch at your desk with poses like Seated Neck Stretches or Seated Marching. This can help alleviate tension and boost energy.

Bedtime Routines:

Wind down with calming poses like Seated Child's Pose or Gentle Seated Forward Fold. Pair these with deep breathing to promote restful sleep.

Chair yoga fits seamlessly into any lifestyle, offering flexibility and convenience while enhancing your overall well-being.

7-Day Beginner's Plan: Daily Routines for Flexibility and Relaxation

This plan introduces you to chair yoga with a focus on building flexibility and relaxation. Each day includes simple routines that gradually increase in intensity while promoting mindfulness and well-being.

Day	Focus	Routine	Duration	Goal
Day 1 ❂	Introduction to Chair Yoga	**- Gentle Wrist Rolls and Hand Stretches** **- Seated Shoulder Rolls** **- Gentle Seated Forward Fold with Breathing**	10–15 minutes	Familiarize yourself with basic poses and focus on gentle movement.
Day 2 ❀	Flexibility for the Upper Body	**- Chair Cat-Cow Stretch** **- Seated Neck and Shoulder Stretches** **- Seated Side Stretches**	15 minutes	Loosen tension in the shoulders, neck, and back while building awareness of your breath.
Day 3 ❀	Core Activation	**- Seated Side Twists for Core Strength** **- Seated Knee-to-Elbow Crunches** **- Core Strengthening Forward Fold**	15–20 minutes	Engage your core muscles gently and improve spinal flexibility.
Day 4 ❦	Lower Body Focus	**- Seated Heel Raises for Calf Toning** **- Seated Pigeon Pose (for Hips)** **- Seated Hamstring Stretch**	15 minutes	Stretch and strengthen your legs, hips, and calves to improve mobility.
Day 5 ❁	Stress Relief and Relaxation	**- Seated Breathing and Visualization** **- Seated Child's Pose** **- Guided Seated Meditation**	10–15 minutes	Cultivate calm and reduce stress with mindfulness and breathing exercises.

| Day
6 | Full-Body Flow | - **Chair Sun Salutation**
- **Chair Warrior II**
- **Gentle Seated Backbend** | 20 minutes | Practice a flowing sequence to stretch and strengthen the entire body. |
| Day
7 | Integration and Reflection | - **Your Favorite Poses (Choose 3–4)**
- **Guided Relaxation with Seated Breathing** | 15 minutes | Reflect on the week, revisit favorite poses, and connect with your breath. |

How to Use This Plan:

- **Consistency Over Perfection:** Stick to the schedule as closely as possible, but don't worry if you need extra rest or modifications.

- **Adjust for Time:** If needed, reduce or extend the session times to fit your schedule.

- **Build a Habit:** Set aside the same time each day for your practice to make it part of your routine.

- **Listen to Your Body:** Skip poses that feel uncomfortable or modify as needed.

30-Day Chair Yoga Challenge (Strength, Weight Loss, and Energy Boost)

This 30-days challenge is designed to improve strength, support weight loss, and boost energy levels. Each week focuses on a specific theme while gradually increasing intensity. By the end of the month, you'll feel stronger, more energized, and confident in your chair yoga practice.

Focus: Strength, Weight Loss, and Energy Boost

Week	Day ❋	Theme	Exercises	Duration	Goal/Focus
Week 1: Flexibility and Relaxation					
	Day 1	Gentle Start	- Seated Shoulder Rolls - Gentle Wrist Rolls and Hand Stretches	15 minutes	Loosen up your shoulders and wrists to release tension.
	Day 2	Deep Breathing Focus	- Gentle Seated Forward Fold with Breathing - Seated Breathing and Visualization	15 minutes	Connect with your breath to reduce stress and improve mindfulness.
	Day 3	Back Stretching	- Chair Cat-Cow Stretch - Gentle Seated Backbend	15 minutes	Relieve back stiffness and enhance spinal flexibility.
	Day 4	Core Awakening	- Core Strengthening Forward Fold - Seated Knee-to-Elbow Crunches	15 minutes	Activate your core gently and improve abdominal strength.
	Day 5	Lower Body Flexibility	- Seated Hamstring Stretch - Seated Pigeon Pose (for Hips)	20 minutes	Stretch tight hamstrings and hips to improve mobility.
	Day	Full-Body	- Seated Sun	20	Flow through gentle

	Day				
	6	Flow	Salutation - Chair Warrior II	minutes	poses to build body awareness and balance.
	Day 7	Restorative Day	- Guided Seated Meditation - Seated Breathing with Visualization	15 minutes	Focus on mindfulness and relaxation to prepare for Week 2.
Week 2: Strength and Weight Loss					
	Day 8	Core Strengthener	- Seated Knee-to-Elbow Crunches - Seated Side Twists for Core Strength - Core Strengthening Forward Fold	15 minutes	Engage and tone your core muscles.
	Day 9	Upper Body Activation	- Chair Arm Circles (Weighted Optional) - Chair Tricep Dips - Seated Boxing Punches	20 minutes	Tone and strengthen your arms and shoulders.
	Day 10	Lower Body Focus	- Seated Heel Raises for Calf Toning - Seated Pigeon Pose (for Hips) - Seated Hamstring Stretch	20 minutes	Boost leg and hip flexibility while improving strength.
	Day 11	Cardio Burn	- Seated Marching with Arm Movements - Chair Jumping Jacks (Arms Only) - Seated Boxing Punches	15–20 minutes	Elevate your heart rate with gentle cardio movements.
	Day 12	Flow and Strength	- Chair Warrior II - Seated Sun Salutation - Seated Side Plank	20 minutes	Combine flowing sequences with strength-building poses.

			Pose (Modified)		
	Day 13 ✺	Relax and Recharge	- Gentle Seated Forward Fold with Breathing - Seated Breathing and Visualization	15 minutes	Focus on mindful relaxation and recovery.
	Day 14 ◗	Reflection and Mindfulness	- Guided Seated Meditation - Chair Cat-Cow Stretch	10–15 minutes	Deepen your connection with mindfulness and breathwork.
Week 3: Energy and Endurance					
	Day 15 ❈	Energizing Flow	- Chair Sun Salutation - Seated Shoulder Rolls - Gentle Seated Backbend	20 minutes	Boost energy with a flowing sequence.
	Day 16 ❧	Core and Balance Focus	- Seated Side Twists for Core Strength - Seated Side Plank Pose (Modified)	15–20 minutes	Improve balance and core stability.
	Day 17 ✿	Lower Body Endurance	- Seated Marching with Arm Movements - Seated Heel Raises for Calf Toning	20 minutes	Build strength and stamina in your lower body.
	Day 18 ✿	Upper Body Focus	- Chair Arm Circles (Weighted Optional) - Chair Tricep Dips - Seated Boxing Punches	20 minutes	Tone and strengthen your upper body muscles.
	Day 19 ✿	Cardio and Energy Boost	- Chair Jumping Jacks (Arms Only) - Seated Marching with Arm Movements	20 minutes	Get your heart pumping with gentle cardio exercises.
	Day	Stretch and	- Seated Pigeon Pose	15–20	Focus on flexibility and

	20 ✸	Relaxation	(for Hips) - Seated Hamstring Stretch - Guided Relaxation with Seated Breathing	minutes	calmness.
	Day 21	Recovery and Reflection	- Guided Seated Meditation - Your Favorite Poses (Choose 3)	15 minutes	Reflect on your progress and focus on your favorite poses.
Week 4: Mastery and Celebration					
	Day 22– 28 ✸	Personalize Your Practice	Each day, combine poses and sequences you've learned to create a 20-minute flow.	20 minutes	Build confidence by creating and practicing a routine that feels good for your body.
	Day 29	Full-Body Celebration	- Chair Sun Salutation - Chair Warrior II - Seated Side Plank Pose (Modified)	20 minutes	Celebrate your progress with a full-body energizing flow.
	Day 30 ✸	Reflection and Gratitude	- Guided Seated Meditation - Seated Breathing and Visualization	15 minutes	Reflect on your journey and celebrate your accomplishments.

Tips for Success:

- 📝 **Track Progress:** Use a journal to note how you feel after each session.

- ✨ **Stay Consistent:** Dedicate the same time each day to your practice.

- 🎉 **Celebrate Wins:** Reward yourself for completing each week!

Part 7: Success Stories

Real-Life Transformations with Chair Yoga ✵

Chair yoga isn't just about stretching or gentle movement—it's a gateway to life-changing benefits for people of all ages and abilities. From regaining mobility to boosting confidence, the real-life stories below show just how transformative this practice can be. Let's dive into a few heartwarming, inspiring journeys that may encourage you to roll out your chair and start your own transformation.

"From Couch to Confident: Lisa's Story"

Lisa, a 54-year-old teacher, struggled with knee pain and low energy after years of sedentary work. Conventional yoga classes felt overwhelming, but chair yoga? It was her perfect match.

✵ **The Turning Point:** Starting with 10-minute sessions, Lisa practiced gentle Seated Marching and Chair Warrior II. Within three weeks, she noticed improved flexibility and less stiffness in her joints.

♡ **Results:**

- Lisa now moves through her day with less pain.
- She's back to gardening—something she hadn't done in years.
- Her energy levels are higher, and she feels more positive.

☞ **Her Tip:** "Consistency matters! Even 5 minutes a day can add up to big changes."

"Regaining Strength After Surgery: Tom's Journey"

After undergoing hip surgery, Tom, a 67-year-old retiree, found it difficult to regain his strength. A friend suggested chair yoga, and it became his secret weapon for recovery.

✵ **The Turning Point:** Chair Sun Salutations and Seated Heel Raises helped Tom rebuild lower body strength without putting pressure on his healing hip.

♡ **Results:**

- Tom's balance improved significantly, giving him confidence to walk unaided.
- He now enjoys daily walks around the park and even plays with his grandkids.
- Chair yoga became a cornerstone of his post-surgery rehabilitation.

☞ **His Tip:** "Don't rush. Listen to your body and celebrate every small step forward!"

"Beating Emotional Eating: Sarah's Transformation"

For Sarah, a 42-year-old graphic designer, stress from work led to emotional eating and weight gain. She turned to chair yoga as a way to manage her stress and break the cycle.

❇ **The Turning Point:** Chair Cat-Cow Stretch paired with Guided Breathing helped Sarah develop mindfulness around her stress triggers.

♀ **Results:**

- She now practices Stress-Relief Flows whenever she feels overwhelmed.
- Sarah lost 15 pounds over 6 months, combining chair yoga with healthier eating habits.
- She feels more in control of her emotions and enjoys a newfound sense of calm.

☞ **Her Tip:** "Use yoga as a pause button for your mind—it's a game-changer!"

"Active at 80: Joan's Success Story"

Joan, an 80-year-old grandmother, thought she was "too old" to start yoga. A local senior center's chair yoga class changed her mind—and her life.

❇ **The Turning Point:** Gentle Wrist Rolls and Seated Shoulder Stretches eased her arthritis pain, while Seated Sun Salutations gave her a gentle energy boost.

♀ **Results:**

- Joan's joint pain has lessened, and her posture has improved.
- She feels more independent, climbing stairs and carrying groceries with ease.
- Chair yoga became a social activity she looks forward to every week.

☞ **Her Tip:** "You're never too old to start. Just show up and enjoy the process."

"Fitting Fitness into a Busy Schedule: Mike's Experience"

Mike, a 36-year-old entrepreneur, struggled to fit exercise into his hectic workdays. Chair yoga became his go-to fitness routine between meetings.

❇ **The Turning Point:** Quick Chair Cardio routines, like Seated Boxing Punches and Chair Jumping Jacks, helped Mike stay active without disrupting his work.

♀ **Results:**

- Mike now completes 15-minute chair yoga sessions daily, even during his lunch break.
- His focus and productivity at work have improved significantly.
- He feels stronger, healthier, and more balanced overall.

☞ **His Tip:** "Chair yoga is flexible enough to fit any schedule—just make it a priority!"

Real people, real results. These testimonials highlight the positive impact chair yoga has had on seniors and beginners, proving that this practice truly is for everyone. Let their words inspire you to take your own first steps (or seated stretches) toward better health and happiness.

Seniors Speak Out

"I feel like I got my life back!"

"Chair yoga has been a blessing for me. At 72, I thought my mobility was gone for good, but the gentle stretches have made my joints feel alive again. I love how easy it is to follow, and I can do it right from my living room. My favorite pose? The Seated Sun Salutation—it feels like I'm welcoming a new day every time I do it!"

— Margaret T., 72, Retired Teacher

"Pain doesn't control me anymore."

"Living with arthritis was exhausting. Chair yoga gave me a way to move without the pain. Simple moves like Gentle Wrist Rolls and Seated Shoulder Stretches have loosened up my joints and made daily tasks easier. I feel stronger and more capable than I have in years!"

— John R., 80, Army Veteran

"It's my new morning ritual."

"I start every morning with 15 minutes of chair yoga, and it has completely changed my outlook on the day. I feel more energized and positive, and I'm even sleeping better. The Guided Seated Meditation at the end of the day is the perfect way to wind down. Who knew something so simple could make such a big difference?"

— Rose M., 67, Retired Librarian

Beginners' Experiences

"I finally found an exercise I enjoy."

"I've always been intimidated by traditional yoga. Chair yoga was a game-changer—it's so approachable and doesn't make me feel out of place. The Seated Marching and Chair Arm Circles are so much fun, and I can feel my strength building without ever stepping foot in a gym!"

— Emma L., 38, Stay-at-Home Mom

"No more excuses!"

"I used to tell myself I didn't have time to work out, but chair yoga fits perfectly into my busy schedule. I squeeze in a 10-minute session during my lunch break, and it helps me stay focused for the rest of the day. I'm already feeling the difference in my energy and posture."

— Mark P., 41, Software Developer

"The perfect recovery tool."

"I was nervous about exercising after my knee surgery, but chair yoga made it easy to ease back into movement. The Seated Heel Raises and Core Strengthening Forward Fold have helped me rebuild strength without overdoing it. I'm so grateful for this gentle yet effective workout!"

— Linda K., 59, Photographer

Conclusion

As we come to the end of this journey, let's take a moment to reflect on all you've achieved and the path that lies ahead. Chair yoga is more than just an exercise; it's a lifestyle that nurtures your body, mind, and spirit.

Reflecting on Your Progress

Think back to where you started—your goals, doubts, and the first steps you took. Now, look at how far you've come. Maybe you feel more flexible, stronger, or less stressed. Perhaps you've discovered moments of peace in your day that weren't there before.

Take pride in every stretch, every breath, and every pose you've practiced. Progress isn't just about physical achievements—it's about showing up for yourself and making your well-being a priority.

Questions for Reflection:

- What changes have you noticed in your body, energy, or mindset?

- What was your favorite part of this journey?

- How has chair yoga influenced other areas of your life?

Write down your thoughts or share them with someone close to you. Celebrating your wins, big or small, reinforces your commitment to long-term well-being.

Maintaining Long-Term Benefits

Chair yoga isn't just a challenge or a one-time journey—it's a sustainable practice that can enhance your life for years to come. Here are some tips to help you maintain and build on your progress:

1. Keep a Regular Schedule

- Set aside a consistent time each day, even if it's just 10 minutes.

- Incorporate chair yoga into daily activities like TV time, work breaks, or your morning routine.

2. Adjust to Your Needs

- Feeling more confident? Add intensity or explore advanced modifications.

- Need something gentler? Focus on relaxation poses and mindfulness exercises.

3. Track Your Progress

- Use the printable tracker or a simple notebook to log your sessions, favorite poses, and how you feel afterward.

- Celebrate milestones like trying a new pose or completing a week of daily practice.

4. Stay Motivated

- Join a local or online chair yoga community for support and inspiration.

- Revisit the testimonials in this guide to remind yourself of the incredible benefits of chair yoga.

5. Pair with Other Healthy Habits

- Combine your practice with a balanced diet, meditation, or light cardio to support your overall wellness.

- Use affirmations to maintain a positive mindset.

A Final Word

Chair yoga has shown you that movement is possible for everyone, no matter your age, fitness level, or limitations. By making this practice a part of your life, you're investing in your health and happiness.

Your journey doesn't end here—it's only just begun. Keep stretching, breathing, and growing. The best version of you is always just one pose away.

Namaste! 🙏